W9-CEJ-053

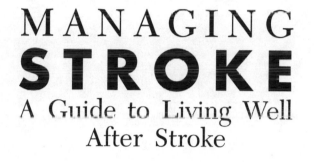

MANAGING
STROKE
A Guide to Living Well
After Stroke

MANAGING
STROKE
A Guide to Living Well After Stroke

Edited by

PAUL R. RAO, Ph.D.
MARK N. OZER, M.D.
JOHN E. TOERGE, D.O.

Foreword by

Don A. Olson, Ph.D.

ABI Professional Publications

Arlington, Virginia

Acknowledgments

I am indebted to Edward A. Eckenhoff, President and CEO of NRH, for helping establish NRH Press. But more importantly, I thank Ed from the bottom of my heart for envisioning and finally building the National Rehabilitation Hospital. The bricks and mortar, bodies and souls and yes, blood, sweat, and tears have melded over these many years to create an incredible experience of "adding life to years" with service, compassion, and pride. The National Rehabilitation Hospital has touched so many and this NRH experience has now resulted in another guide to living well, this volume for persons with stroke.

I would like to thank my co-editors, Dr. John Toerge and Dr. Mark Ozer, for assisting in this compendium for consumers and more importantly for playing significant roles in my career at NRH. Dr. John gambled fifteen years ago and went with a novice Ph.D. and rookie manager to become NRH's inaugural Director of the Speech Language Pathology Service. I have loved the challenges of patient care, teaching, management, research and writing that the NRH has afforded me. John gave me a shot and I took it. Dr. Ozer and I co directed the Stroke Recovery Program for nearly a decade and under his tutelage, I became more convinced than ever that "patient as partner" was the path to recovering from a stroke.

I must thank each member of Team NRH who took the time to share their expertise on rehabilitation by contributing to this book, while doing all of their other jobs at NRH. Dr. Brendan Conroy, the current medical director of NRH's Stroke Recovery Program, read the entire text for consistency and accuracy and provided many useful edits. Part IV of the book is actually the highlight for me since it is composed of the stories of people with stroke who have shared their hopes and dreams, home-grown remedies, fears and frustrations, and success stories.

I thank these folks for the guts to share openly what each has learned as he or she underwent the art and science of rehabilitation. I am particularly indebted to Craig and Carol, Nancy and Nate, Bill and Pat, and John for their candor, courage and friendship.

I would like to thank Robert Hartman for assisting with the logistics of this second volume of NRH Press and for the support and "can-do" spirit of Arthur Brown, the publisher. Peggie Matthews and Beverly Morris were key to getting the book word processed and printed. . .again in addition to their many other duties. *The Consumer Guide for People with Stroke*, which was the precursor of the present volume, was co-authored with Michelle Rives. Michelle's initial work and ideas on health insurance and consumer choice have made this new "consumer guide" on stroke much more doable and relevant.

Finally, for all those late nights and weekends when I was either editing or writing, I want to thank the love of my life, Martina, for her patience, understanding, and support . . . I owe you big time.

Paul Rao, Ph.D.
Editor

Contributors

Christine Baron, M.A., C.C.C.
Co-Director, Stroke Recovery
    Program
Manager, Speech Language
    Pathology
National Rehabilitation Hospital
Washington D.C.

Philip Beatty, M.A.
Research Associate
NRH Research Center
National Rehabilitation Hospital
Washington D.C.

Helen Bozzo, C.R.R.N.
Manager, NRH/Visiting Nurses
    Association
Home Care Program
Washington D.C.

Carol Bullard-Bates, Ph.D.
Neuropsychologist
National Rehabilitation Hospital
Washington D.C.

Martha Carroll, M.S., PT
Physical Therapy Clinical
    Supervisor
National Rehabilitation Hospital
Washington D.C.

Carrie Clawson, B.S., OTR/L,
Stafff Occupational Therapist
National Rehabilitation Hospital
Washington D.C.

Brendan E. Conroy, M.D.
Medical Director, Stroke
    Recovery Program
National Rehabilitation Hospital
Washington D.C.

Gerben DeJong, Ph.D.
Director, NRH Research Center
National Rehabilitation Hospital
Washington D.C.

Mathew Elrod, M.Ed., PT
Staff Physical Therapist
National Rehabilitation Hospital
Washington D.C.

Judie Gray, C.A.N.P., M.S.N.
Nurse Practitioner
Stroke Recovery Program
National Rehabilitation Hospital
Washington D.C.

Jennifer Hendricks, L.I.C.S.W.
Manager, Care Co-ordination
National Rehabilitation Hospital
Washington D.C.

Richard Keller, B.S.
Clinical Rehabilitation Engineer
National Rehabilitation Hospital
Washington D.C.

Audrey Kinsella, M.S.
Research Librarian Consultant
National Rehabilitation Hospital
Washington D.C.

Brenda McCall-Russell, C.R.R.N.
Nursing Education
National Rehabilitation Hospital
Washington D.C.

Fatemeh Milani, M.D.
Physiatrist, Stroke Recovery
  Program
National Rehabilitation Hospital
Washington D.C.

John Noiseux, M.S., ATP
Assistive Technology Specialist
National Rehabilitation Hospital
Washington D.C.

Mark N. Ozer, M.D.
Director, Program for Clinical
  Excellence
National Rehabilitation Hospital
Washington D.C.

Paul R. Rao, Ph.D.
Vice President, Clinical Services,
  Quality Improvement, &
  Corporate Compliance
National Rehabilitation Hospital
Washington D.C.

Michael Rosen, Ph.D.
Director, Rehabilitation
  Engineering Service
National Rehabilitation Hospital
Washington D.C.

Trudy Sellman, C.R.R.N.
Primary Nurse II
Washington Hospital Center
Washington D.C.

John E. Toerge, D.O.
Senior Vice President, Medical
  Affairs and Medical Director
National Rehabilitation Hospital
Washington D.C.

Cheryl Trepagnier, Ph.D.
Senior Research Consultant,
  Rehabilitation Engineering
  Service
National Rehabilitation Hospital
Washington D.C.

Gretchen Braun Vidergar, M.A., OTR/L
Senior Occupational Therapist
National Rehabilitation Hospital
Washington D.C.

Contents

Foreword

DON A. OLSON

Today's health and rehabilitation practices call for a new paradigm. New goals for the healthcare professional include understanding the need for prevention programs, developing innovative ways to encourage empowerment of the consumer, and facilitating re-integration into the community of choice. *Managing Stroke: A Guide to Living Well After A Stroke* promotes this paradigm shift for the person recovering from stroke. It is an easy-to-read, comprehensive, and practical approach to a challenging and overwhelming problem for thousands of people. It also provides information for making the patient and their family true members of the rehabilitation team.

The goal of rehabilitation has always been to enhance the quality of life for those affected by the consequences of a stroke. As professionals, we have always known how to work as a team to achieve this goal and have brought many areas of professional interest together which are required for the practice of a program in stroke rehabilitation. The field of rehabilitation for persons with physical disabilities has made significant progress as a medical, allied health, and nursing specialty. This progress has been greater in the past few years because of the incorporation of the person recovering from a stroke and his/her family into the rehabilitation planning process.

One of the most overlooked aspects of rehabilitation is the "experience of the stroke" as perceived and described by the patient. An understanding by the clinicians of the prospective of the patient and his or her family is essential to providing effective care and to addressing the needs of the person recovering from a stroke. Patients and families have much to teach us, and we have much to learn from them. Organizations such as the American Heart Association, the National Stroke Association, and the National Aphasia Association have provided materials on a regular basis to patients and families. We as professionals in these and other organizations are now seeing the need for expanded patient/family education resources to complement the medical, allied health and nursing approaches that we use in physical medicine and rehabilitation. In the future, we will be seeing a greater number of materials developed which will empower the individual with a stroke to solve many of his/her own problems and to select the options that meet his/her own special needs. This book can be used as a resource for that very purpose.

The Independent Living Movement has been another option for both the rehabilitation professional and the consumer. These consumer run, organized, and staffed programs help to make rehabilitation more relevant and are a major partner and player in the total scope of rehabilitation today. It is important that these programs are integrated into both the lives of the recovering disabled individual and facilities offering rehabilitation services. The goal of integration of persons with disabilities into the community is equal to that of rehabilitation medicine. The Independent Living Movement's desire and need for education and training materials for wellness, housing, transportation, legal issues and all of life's challenges support the content of this book.

A major challenge for today's healthcare worker, patient, and family has been the shortened rehabilitation stay in the rehabilitation facility. Rehabilitation is basically an educational process, where the patient learns how to compensate and manage his own disabilities. Shorter stays in a rehabilitation facility impact the amount of education and training that can be undertaken during the rehabilitation process. Supplementary approaches to education and training needs for consumers are mandatory for successful rehabilitation. Thus, the need for more education and training materials is especially critical.

The authors, mostly taken from one of the nation's leading rehabilitation hospitals, provide important clinical insights to help to close the gap between academic research, clinical experiences, and solving life's problems. The involvement of former patients and individuals recovering from stroke is a great strength of this book. It, therefore, provides a resource – not only for the professionals, but also for persons recovering from a stroke and their family members.

Director
Dixon Education and Training Center
Rehabilitation Institute of Chicago

Associate Professor
Departments of Physical Medicine and Rehabilitation and Neurology
Northwestern University Medical School
Chicago, Illinois

Editor
Topics In Stroke Rehabilitation

Introduction

In 1996, the National Rehabilitation Hospital (NRH) Research Center published a *Consumer Guide for People with Stroke* with support from the National Institute on Disability and Rehabilitation Research. Dramatic changes in the health care and rehabilitation environment during the past few years have warranted the publication of this second, expanded edition of the guide: *Managing Stroke: A Guide to Living Well.* Among the changes that have occurred since publication of the original guide was the passage of the Balanced Budget Act of 1997 (Public Law 105-33). This legislation has had a profound effect on long-term care, and in the year 2000 will result in a prospective payment system for rehabilitation reimbursement. In addition, consumers need current, practical information about how to navigate the healthcare system and will need to understand the new, federally mandated patients' rights legislation.

Managing Stroke is designed to arm the person with stroke with the knowledge needed to cope with the aftermath of stroke. Consistent with NRH's credo of "Adding Life to Years," it is our hope that this guide will enable readers to live productively and fully, to be as healthy as possible, and to fulfill their personal goals and aspirations. This guide is written to educate readers about living well after stroke. It suggests a novel way to participate in decision making and the ongoing revision of one's life plans. This "patient as partner" approach is an essential part of medical rehabilitation and an overarching theme in this book.

Managing Stroke provides a comprehensive overview of issues associated with the medical, psychological, financial, and many other challenges of living with stroke. Written by 16 medical rehabilitation authorities, this guide distills the wealth of knowledge on stroke and rehabilitation that has been developed during the past decade. The book is written in four principal parts.

Part One of *Managing Stroke* is entitled "Facts and Myths in Dealing with Stroke and its Aftermath." The lead chapter in this section provides important information about stroke, rehabilitation, and the expected outcomes of rehabilitation. Several subsequent chapters, written in a question-and-answer format, address the typical challenges faced by the stroke survivor and family—from dealing with the shock of admission to an acute-care hospital for a 'brain attack' to selecting a rehabilitation facility to community re-entry following rehabilitation. The final chapter in Part One provides an overview of the types and sources of public and private health insurance. In addition, the section on stroke outcomes provides a user-friendly primer on the current thinking about attainable outcomes after stroke. After reading this section, the person with stroke will know what questions to ask and where to find the answers to those questions.

Part Two, entitled "Planning and Carrying Out Solutions to Post-Stroke Problems," includes a chapter on the planning process that identifies the problems. It then discusses the management of each problem in a structured and empowering fashion. The problems addressed include bowel and bladder management, the use of blood thinners, and coping with high blood pressure, high cholesterol, and diabetes. As a result of becoming familiar with this section, the stroke survivor who is experiencing one of these problems will better understand the problem, and, more importantly, will know how to manage the problem in partnership with his or her healthcare provider.

Part Three, entitled "Medical Rehabilitation: The Professionals and Approaches to Coping with Stroke," contains chapters on post-stroke challenges that are managed by the patient in conjunction with rehabilitation professionals. Among the issues addressed are communication and swallowing problems, daily living activities (such as dressing, cooking, driving, walking, and using equipment), emotional problems common in coping with stroke, use of technology in the home and other environments, and problems in adapting to and living well at home. Also included is a discussion of the Internet as it relates to stroke. This chapter discusses everything from getting on a stroke listserv to surfing the World Wide Web to find answers to pressing questions. After reading this section, the consumer with stroke will better understand the purpose and goals of rehabilitation, as well as strategies that have proven successful in overcoming post-stroke problems. Also the consumer will be equipped to begin surfing the 'net' for answers and support.

Part Four, entitled "Consumers Speak Out," presents vignettes about individuals who provide eloquent, often heroic testimony to the many ways people have prevailed in the face of ongoing disability. For example, the reader meets Craig, who was mute following a catastrophic stroke and later became fully and gainfully employed with a major U.S. airline. This section celebrates the idea of "adding life to years," as seen through the hearts, minds, and souls of persons with stroke and their families and friends. After reading these poignant stories about individuals who have fought against odds to "strike back at stroke," the reader will feel less alone and more empowered to face life's challenges.

The appendix to *Managing Stroke*, entitled "Post-Stroke Resources," includes a glossary of stroke-related terms, a consumer checklist of important quality characteristics and criteria for choosing a rehabilitation program, a comprehensive listing of stroke-related resources, and a list of informational references and additional readings on each of the chapter topics included in the book. After reading this section, stroke survivors and family members will better understand some of the terms they may hear, know what questions to ask when evaluating a prospective rehabilitation program, know how to access resources in the community, and be more aware of useful print and electronic information resources that might be helpful in better understanding and coping with stroke

Paul R. Rao, Ph.D.,
Mark N. Ozer, M.D.,
John E. Toerge, D.O.,
Editors

MANAGING
STROKE

A Guide to Living Well
After Stroke

—1—
Background on Stroke and Rehabilitation

PAUL R. RAO
BRENDAN E. CONROY
JOHN E. TOERGE

Selecting a medical rehabilitation program after you, a member of your family, or a close friend has had a stroke may be one of the most important and difficult medical decisions you will ever make. Therefore, it is very important that your decision be based on the most complete and up-to-date information available, especially now, when the health care system is changing so rapidly.

Unfortunately, you must usually decide about stroke rehabilitation when you do not have the luxury of time to conduct a lengthy survey of rehabilitation programs. Typically, a person who has had a stroke is rushed to the nearest emergency room and admitted to an acute-care hospital where he or she stays for approximately one week. Most people in stable medical condition are ready to be transferred to another type of facility within the first week after their stroke. This leaves little time to consider all available options and to answer all of the important questions about where to go for medical rehabilitation.

Within a few days after the stroke, someone at the acute-care hospital will speak to the family or other loved ones about beginning the challenging decision of where to go next. Usually, a spouse, an adult child, or another family member becomes the key decision maker to determine the most appropriate and affordable rehabilitation for the person with stroke. Thus, this person is asked to select a rehabilitation program in a time of crisis, when he or she and the person with stroke are more concerned about immediate medical and personal issues than about where to go for rehabilitation.

1

> *KNOWLEDGE is Power!*
> *The more you understand about your medical condition and*
> *the available kinds of rehabilitation programs, the more*
> *involved you can be in making decisions about your stroke*
> *rehabilitation.*

HOW CAN THIS BOOK HELP ME TO STRIKE BACK AT STROKE?

This book was written to serve as a guide to living well following a stroke. First, it explains briefly what a stroke is and some of the problems stroke causes. In addition, Part I describes the choices that are available for stroke rehabilitation and how health insurance affects those choices. Part II describes the planning and carrying out of the solutions to post-stroke problems. In Part III, the authors attempt to explain what rehabilitation is and what can be expected from it. Part IV is a forum for persons with stroke to share their post-stroke insights, ideas and accomplishments. Finally, there are helpful appendices located at the back of this guide: a checklist for evaluating stroke rehabilitation programs, a listing of stroke resources, and a glossary that defines the terms shown in **boldfaced** type throughout the guide.

ABOUT STROKE

The first step in dealing with the aftermath of stroke is understanding what has happened. In this section the reader will learn what a stroke is, how it affects the brain, and the kinds of problems it can cause.

What is a Stroke?

Stroke is a type of brain injury caused by a sudden interruption of the blood flow to the brain. An interruption in blood flow can occur when a blood vessel is either blocked (a blood clot) or bursts (a cerebral hemorrhage). When blood cannot reach the brain, brain cells become deprived of oxygen and die and cause damage to that area of the brain.

- Stroke is the third leading cause of death in the United States and the number one cause of adult disability.
- Half a million people each year have strokes, and three million Americans are living with stroke-related problems today.
- The risk of stroke more than doubles with each decade after age 55. Seventy-two percent of all people with stroke are age 65 or older.
- African Americans have a 60 percent greater risk of having a stroke than Caucasians.
- Men have a greater risk of stroke than do women.
- Certain medical conditions are major risk factors for having a stroke. These include: high blood pressure; transient ischemic attacks (TIAs), also called stroke warning signs; previous stroke; heart disease (especially atrial fibrillation); diabetes; and carotid artery disease.
- People with a family history of stroke and people who smoke also have a greater risk for stroke.

How Does Stroke Affect the Brain?

When an area of the brain is damaged by stroke, body functions controlled by the damaged area no longer work as before. For example, if the front portion of the brain is damaged, the face, hand, or arm might become paralyzed. If the back portion of the brain is damaged, a loss of vision might occur. There are four areas of brain function that can be affected by stroke:

- motor control (such as movement of an arm or leg)
- sensation (such as touch, hearing or vision)
- communication and intelligence (such as talking or thinking)
- personality and character (such as moods or emotions)

A person who has had a stroke may experience a single problem, or a combination of problems in any or all of the four areas of brain function listed above. Many times, a stroke on one side of the brain affects

functions on the opposite side of the body. For example, a stroke on
the left side of the brain might cause a person to become paralyzed on
the right side of the body, become blind in the right half of vision,
have problems talking, and have inappropriate outbursts of laughter
or crying.

What Kinds of Problems Does Stroke Cause?

Stroke is a serious medical condition; yet everyone is affected differently and to different degrees. No two strokes are alike. Stroke can affect many brain functions and cause many different kinds of medical
and neurological problems, some of which are described below.

Medical Problems

- Swallowing problems, called **dysphagia**, are common after
  stroke. Problems with swallowing may result in food getting in
  the lungs, which in turn may cause pneumonia. Sometimes swallowing difficulties are so serious after a stroke that a doctor must
  insert a feeding tube through the patient's nose, neck or stomach
  to prevent dehydration and malnutrition.
- Bladder control problems, also called incontinence, occur in
  nearly half of all people with stroke. Bladder control often returns during the stroke recovery period.
- Bowel function problems, such as fecal incontinence or constipation, occur in nearly a third of all people with stroke, but usually clear up within a couple of weeks after the stroke.
- Pressure sores, or decubitus ulcers, occur when the person with
  stroke is unable to relieve pressure on certain body parts when
  sitting or lying in bed. This pressure can result in a serious skin
  breakdown possibly requiring reparative surgery.
- Falls are a common problem among people with stroke. Falls
  may result from other stroke-related problems, such as confusion, loss of balance and coordination, paralysis, and communication problems preventing one from asking for help when
  needed.
- Blood clots that form in the veins and travel to the lungs are a
  major cause of illness, and sometimes death, among people with
  stroke.

- Restlessness and altered sleep patterns may result from the effects of stroke and from the different routine of the hospital environment. Lack of adequate sleep can seriously interfere with a person's ability to recover.

Neurological Problems

- Movement and feeling problems, also called motor and sensory problems, are the most common problems following stroke. People with stroke may become paralyzed; experience weakness; or have decreased sensation in the hand, arm or leg that could affect activities such as standing, sitting, walking, feeding, bathing, grooming, and other **activities of daily living (ADLs)**.
- Speech and language problems occur in more than 40 percent of people with stroke. **Aphasia, dysarthria,** and **apraxia** are words that soon become familiar to families of people who have communication problems following stroke.
- Thinking and perception problems, also called cognitive and perceptual problems, are typical among people with stroke. People with stroke often experience changes in their mental abilities, such as problems with attention and memory, or changes in their perception of the world around them, for example, **neglect,** such as ignoring sensory information coming from the right or left side of their body.
- Depression and other emotional problems are also common. People with stroke may feel hopeless and pessimistic, and may experience changes in their eating or sleeping patterns due to depression.

ABOUT MEDICAL REHABILITATION

Many of us think of medical rehabilitation in the same way we think of other medical treatment: If you have a broken leg, you get it set, let it heal in a cast for six weeks, and are then ready to walk again. This is not the case with medical rehabilitation. There is no magic pill or medical procedure that can help a paralyzed person suddenly walk again. Rehabilitation requires much patience, motivation, hard work, and time. Therefore, after a stroke, you must put aside notions of medical "cures" and think in terms of "relearning old skills" such as how to walk and talk, and "learning new skills," in order to resume life despite the stroke. In this section you will learn about medical rehabilitation: what it is, what it can do for you, and what you and your family must do to make the most of your rehabilitation.

What is Medical Rehabilitation?

Rehabilitation adds life *to years!*

Medical rehabilitation is a specialty dedicated to reducing physical and mental problems, restoring previous abilities, and returning people to their lives after injury or illness. Rehabilitation uses a carefully planned program to help regain the ability to function as independently as possible at home, at work, and in the community.

Medical rehabilitation involves learning to manage one's life again, despite any limitations that result from stroke. The primary aim of medical rehabilitation is to help one achieve the best possible **quality of life**. This means reducing any physical or psychological problems one may have and returning the patient to the community. To reach these goals, the family must be involved throughout the entire rehabilitation process from setting goals to planning and participating in treatment.

The earlier rehabilitation begins, the more likely one is to regain the ability to function and return to a productive and satisfying life. With hard work, commitment, and proper care, even people with serious stroke-related problems can become independent and functional again.

Does Everyone Who Has a Stroke Need Medical Rehabilitation?

For every 100 people with stroke, 10 recover without any rehabilitation and 10 others have such serious problems that they cannot benefit from rehabilitation at all. The remaining 80, however, can benefit from some sort of rehabilitative program.

What Can Rehabilitation Do About Problems Caused By Stroke?

The goal of rehabilitation is to help the patient reach the highest possible level of independence. Rehabilitation does this by closing the gap between the ability to function independently (that is, **functional ability**) and the challenges of the environment. This gap can be closed by:

- enhancing your functional ability through rehabilitation **services** such as physical, occupational, and speech therapy;
- providing **assistive equipment** such as wheelchairs, braces, walkers, and speech aids in order to close the gap between functional ability and environment;
- reducing barriers in the environment through **environmental supports**, such as wider doorways, ramps, or elevators.

Here is an example to explain further what this means. Imagine a scale from zero to 100 where zero represents total dependence and 100 represents total independence. A superhero who can leap tall buildings and flies through the sky might function at 100, but the rest of us fall somewhere below 100 on this "scale of independence." We depend on assistive equipment (such as eyeglasses and hearing aids) and environmental supports (such as stairs, elevators, and automobiles) to deal with day-to-day living and the barriers around us. While a superhero does not need any kind of support to conquer the world around him, people with disabilities may need *extra* support to close the gap between functional ability and the barriers in the environment.

"Medical rehabilitation is the science and art of helping people who survive traumatic injury and potentially disabling disease to lead functional and productive lives."

Medical Rehabilitation Education Foundation

Problems a Person with Stroke Might Experience

Stroke-related problems can range from mild to significant in three different areas:

- Impairments: Problems of organ functions, such as muscular systems (paralysis), nervous systems (sensory loss), or language systems (aphasia).
- Activities (formerly termed "Disabilities"): Problems of human functions, such as walking, self-care, emotional control, seeing, thinking, and communicating.
- Participation (formerly termed "Handicap"): Problems externally imposed by society, such as environmental barriers, negative stereotypes, and fear of people who seem different. Can you participate in society and conduct all of the activities to which you "were" accustomed?

How Can Rehabilitation Help the Individual?

As mentioned above, rehabilitation is not meant to be a "cure," nor does it aim to reduce or repair physical **impairments** (problems of organ functions), such as paralysis. Instead, rehabilitation works to improve your ability to perform **activities** and reduce **disabilities** (problems of human functions) that result from impairments (such as not being able to walk). This is accomplished by enhancing functional ability, providing assistive equipment, and providing environmental supports. For example, if one is paralyzed as a result of a stroke, the patient may receive physical therapy services to improve balance and muscle strength, as well as assistive equipment (such as a cane or wheelchair) to increase independence. When the rehabilitation is complete and the patient is able to get around independently with a cane or a wheelchair, the disability will have been reduced considerably.

Rehabilitation is also directed at increasing participation in society by reducing **handicaps** (problems caused by the environment), such as steps that create a barrier for a person in a wheelchair. One might define a handicap as a barrier, or a limitation of choice. These problems are often the most critical for people with stroke. For example, you might know someone who has a mild disability such as a mild stuttering problem that has become a significant handicap because of a refusal to talk on the phone for fear of stuttering. On the other hand, a person with stroke might have a significant disability such as an inability to talk. The inability might be only a mild handicap because he or she communicates his or her needs by using hand gestures or an alphabet board.

Immediately after a stroke, one might feel quite handicapped because one cannot do everything as before or cannot participate in society as before. However, with the assistance of family members, friends, doctors, therapists, nurses, and others, the patient will learn new ways to walk, talk, dress, and, in general, become less handicapped and more able to participate in daily living activities!

Recovery From Stroke: Functional Outcomes

Since the mid 80s, rehabilitation providers have been gathering patient "outcome" data in an attempt to improve rehabilitation programs. The idea is to determine what worked well in rehab and what didn't work so well. One might hear the term Functional Independence Measure or FIM. The term refers to an outcome measurement scale. The FIM is a tool of rehabilitation therapists, nurses, and doctors to measure limitations of the person with stroke. These abilities include walking, talking, eating and others. The FIM scores, based on a 7 point scale, range from a score of 1 indicating that the patient is judged to be totally disabled to 7 indicating that the patient is able to perform a skill normally. The FIM rating then consists of 18 individual "snapshots" of function at three critical points in the rehabilitation process: when the patient is admitted to the rehab hospital or unit, when the patient is discharged from the rehab hospital or unit, and then finally at three months after discharge. Thus the rehab team knows how the person with stroke was doing on admission, at discharge, and then 90 days later in the community. The therapists speak of a FIM gain to mean the number of FIM points of improvement during the rehab stay. These FIM ratings have been gathered on all acute rehab patients for the last 15 years, so there is a gold mine of "outcomes" data, and that data can be used to make predictions about how the "average" patient with stroke will do. The rehab professionals now have a pretty good idea of what the typical rehabilitation hospital experience will be and what a patient can reasonably expect from his or her stay in the rehabilitation facility. The average stay for a person with stroke in a rehab hospital or unit is about 21 days. Recovery from stroke has a slow but fairly reliable progression. 85% of stroke survivors are able to walk again during the first six months, although a cane might be needed. Swallowing generally returns to near-normal, and the person can eat regular food again. For most stroke patients, control of the bowel and bladder returns, as does the ability to bathe and dress and to think clearly and safely. Research shows that stroke patients who are transferred to acute rehabilitation centers get better faster, go home sooner, and have more comprehensive home-therapy services than do those who go to a sub-acute rehabilitation center or nursing home. As a matter of fact, approximately four out of five stroke patients admitted to a rehab unit or hospital will return to their home and the remaining one out of five will go to a nursing home. It is difficult to predict how much normal strength and co-ordination will return in an affected hand. Recovery from aphasia, the language disorder, is also quite variable. The positive thing about stroke is that generally, patients get better . . . they don't stay the same or get worse as in some other neurological illnesses. Neurologists tend to say that recovery from a stroke happens mostly in the first three to six months, but most stroke rehabilitation professionals say they see their patients continue to make gains in independence for several years following stroke. Recovery is certainly not "finished" just because a magic six months have passed since the "brain attack."

Life After Rehabilitation

Rehabilitation is a process that takes time, hard work and patience. But once rehabilitation is complete, the process of living with stroke begins more earnestly. One needs to resume life without continuous, daily backup from therapists and other rehabilitation professionals. As this process begins, keep in mind that after a stroke there comes a time when recovery slows down and gains in functional ability become smaller. At this point, the focus changes to quality of life and less on recovery. One way to enhance quality of life is to look for activities that are fun and stimulating. A good place to start is participating in support groups. There one can meet people who are engaged in positive experiences. For older people, this might mean participating in outings organized by the American Association of Retired Persons (AARP) or local senior centers.

Because stroke affects more people over the age of 65 than younger people, returning to work may not be an important goal for some people with stroke. Therefore, the same advice that a retirement counselor would give to new retirees is also appropriate for many older people with stroke. There are many stories of people taking up new challenges, such as golf or gardening, after a stroke. Others choose to become involved in community volunteer activities, such as at the local library, or to become active in the local stroke club. Yes, there is life after rehabilitation, but much of the responsibility for the *quality* of that life lies with the stroke patient, the care giver, and the family—not with your rehabilitation team.

Remember that stroke is a family illness, and, because of that, "quality of life" means quality of life for the patient, care giver, and everyone else in the family circle. Community resources are available to find answers and support. Through the local **stroke club**, one meets others with stroke who have moved on with their lives and are willing to share a point of view, a helping hand, an encouraging work, or an honest assessment. This book includes a section called "Stroke Resources" that gives the addresses and phone numbers of the American Heart Association, the National Stroke Association, and other stroke-related organizations providing additional information to help coping with stroke and its life-changing, though hopeful, aftermath. Many of these organizations have local chapters. You are not alone. Nearly three million Americans now confront challenges similar to those you are facing and are discovering that there is "life after rehabilitation." It is up to you to write the next chapter

> *"The earlier rehabilitation begins, the better the results. While acute care saves lives, medical rehabilitation determines quality of life and future employability."*
>
> Medical Rehabilitation Education Foundation

Young People and Stroke

Stroke in young people is not common, but it is traumatic. Young people with stroke have special needs and concerns that can be quite different from those of older people. Issues related to sexuality and employability are particularly important concerns for young people with stroke. Twenty years ago, there was little discussion of sexuality with people with stroke or with their partners. Neither was vocational rehabilitation considered an option. Today, however, there are many resources available to help young people with stroke to get the answers and help they need on issues of sexuality, family and child care, employment and other concerns. Stroke clubs and support groups organized specifically for young people can provide answers and encouragement from other young people who have experienced or are currently experiencing the same feelings and frustrations. Young people with stroke can also return to gainful employment. The Americans with Disabilities Act (ADA) now provides the force of federal law to prevent discrimination against people with disabilities in the workplace. The ADA also requires employers to make "reasonable accommodations" to assist disabled persons in returning to their jobs. For more information about local stroke clubs and support groups for young people or about employment options, talk with the rehabilitation professionals on your team or contact the organizations listed in the "Stroke Resources" section of this guide.

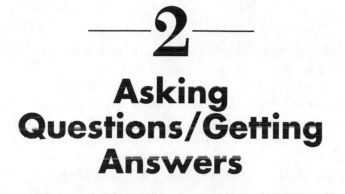

2

Asking Questions/Getting Answers

MARK N. OZER
PAUL RAO
BRENDAN CONROY

ASKING YOUR QUESTIONS/GETTING ANSWERS

This chapter will review the following questions you could have asked and help you define any other questions you might want to ask:

- What happened when I had a stroke?
- What is a stroke?
- What happens next?
- What can cause illness?
- Where is the stroke ?
- What kind of stroke was it?
- How severe is the stroke?
- What caused the stroke?
- How can I prevent another stroke?
- Why would a young person have a stroke?
- What can happen next in getting back to life again?

ACUTE HOSPITAL PHASE

The goal of this first part of the chapter is to answer questions about the stroke that has occurred. You can check off the questions you need to ask on the list above. By the end of this section, you should be able to know what might have caused the stroke and, what could be done to make another stroke less likely. You should also be able to know where the stroke occurred, such as what part of the brain was affected, why certain tests were done, and what medical problems you should ask the physician. At the end of this part, you can find a list of the questions answered in this section, then you can once again check off the questions you have had answered and identify any other questions you may still want to ask. The questions you have during the first week after a stroke are different from those you may ask later. The first questions asked by the patient or the family are usually answered within the first day. The answers need to be available right away. Many questions are asked the first week after the stroke but the answers may come only with time.

How Do I Know I Had a Stroke?

One man had a choking spell when some fluid went down the wrong way. He had been fine just before. His wife noticed that the left side of his face seemed funny. She thought immediately, "My God, he has had a stroke!" The ambulance was called and although he walked out to the door, by the time he had reached the hospital, the entire left side of his body had been affected. How did she know he had a stroke? What are the signs of stroke? What would you do if you had those warning signs?

Another person with a stroke felt some tingling in the arm on one side of her body. It cleared up after a few minutes. She did nothing about the "tingling" and began to get ready for work. She called her office to inform them she did not feel well. Later that day, she began to feel heaviness throughout her arm and leg on one side. By the time she was brought to the hospital, it was finally clear to her that she was having a stroke.

One common characteristic of a stroke or a cerebrovascular accident (CVA) is the loss of control of one side of the body. Usually there is involvement of the face, arm, and leg. There may be loss of vision of the same side. Sensation is frequently affected as well as control of actions. It is rare to feel any pain except possibly a headache. One very important and noticeable change is in the ability to communicate. This communication problem is frequently associated with injury to

Table 2.1 Warning Signs of Stroke

- Sudden numbness or weakness in the face, arm or leg, especially on one side of the body;
- Difficulty speaking or trouble understanding speech;
- Difficulty swallowing;
- Sudden severe headaches with no apparent cause;
- Sudden dizziness, trouble walking, or loss of balance or coordination;
- Episodes of double vision or suddenly blurred or decreased vision, particularly in one eye.

the left side of the brain affecting the right side of the body. Trouble with swallowing and slurring of speech may occur with injury to either side of the brain or the brain stem. The patient might experience episodes of double vision and dizziness like that of sea sickness (see Table 2.1 Warning Signs of Stroke). It is important to act on these warnings. There is increasing evidence that a stroke attack (or "brain attack") should be considered a medical emergency. It has become increasingly important for persons to know these warning signs and to act on them to seek medical help as soon as possible. It is expected also that many more treatments will become available for early treatment of person experiencing a stroke. The term "attack" is being used to convey the urgent need for quick response—a word choice that has proven so helpful in reducing the effects of heart "attacks."

What is a Stroke?

The character of the stroke in its very word indicates a "bolt from the blue," a sudden change. The suddenness of the change one experiences comes from the exquisite sensitivity of nerve cells in the brain to any lack of food. To keep working, the brain cells need a major part of the oxygen in the blood cells and the energy in the form of sugar carried in the blood. Even momentary reduction in this food can cause injury and death to the cells. Injury to the brain cells can occur because of hemorrhage (bleeding) into the brain or blockage of the blood supply. However, some of the injured cells may not be completely destroyed. There is time to save the cells that are not totally destroyed. A brief window of time exists when, if something is done, those partially injured cells may be rescued from ultimate destruction. The goal is to seek help within a three hour opportunity to save a substantial number of nerve cells. The fewer cells destroyed, the less severe is the eventual effect on the person's function. Whether there is actual injury and destruction of nerve cells depends upon the ability of the brain cells to get blood supplied from elsewhere. One opportunity lies in neighboring blood vessels expanding to take over to provide sustenance to the area deprived of its customary blood supply. One reason that strokes tend to occur in the elderly is that as one gets older and the walls of arteries become hardened, even blood vessels nearby may not be able to respond as quickly to a blockage in any one of the vessels.

Another opportunity is to use a drug to dissolve the clot that has blocked the blood coming to the injured area (rTPA, see glossary). If the clot is dissolved, blood can once again provide sustenance to the nerve cells. If given soon enough, a portion of the partially injured nerve cells can be saved from dying. Another opportunity to rescue some of the nerve cells not totally destroyed is now being discovered by the use of various other medications. The effect of the partial death of these cells is for the membranes surrounding the cells to no longer carry out their function of maintaining the correct environment for ongoing metabolism. There is a breakdown in the mineral content of the cell, and with that there is further disintegration. For example, too much calcium is allowed into the cell by the damaged membrane and this worsens the injury. One new drug used is a calcium blocker, such as nimodipine, to keep out the extra calcium.

Another problem is that injured cells release all their contents. Aspartate and glutamate are excitatory neuro-transmitters that nerve cells use in tiny doses to talk to each other. When a large amount of aspartate and glutamate is released suddenly, it can kill nearby cells. Another new type of drug is given to protect nearby cells from the excess aspartate and glutamate floating around. Other drugs keep blood vessels in the damaged area from tightening up or constricting in the presence of these excitatory chemicals.

Another medical treatment option is for a radiologist to puncture the skin of the neck or groin, push a very long hollow wire into the blood stream and float the tip of the wire up into the person's head to the place where a clot has stopped the blood flow. A clot dissolving medicine urokinase is released to try and restore the blood flow. Urokinase and rTPA, known as "clot busters," have reduced the amount of disability of many people with stroke.

Currently, one area of intensive study is the value of various medications in helping to counteract this shift of minerals. The availability of medication for this purpose also makes it critical to seek help immediately after the onset of stroke, before its too late and permanent brain damage has occurred.

What is Going to Happen Next?

Is the patient going to live or die ? This urgent question can more reliably be answered during the next 72 hours when the effects of the stroke may be at their greatest. The most serious problem that can cause early death is the effect of increased pressure within the skull due to hemorrhage or increase in the fluid content of the brain. Bleeding into the brain causes injury to the brain cells where the bleeding occurs. In addition, swelling of the brain, called edema, is caused by the reaction of the brain cells injured by the stroke. The injured cells lose their ability to maintain proper membrane function. Fluid enters the weakened cells and causes them to swell. The presence of injury then causes swelling throughout the brain and brings about further injury of additional brain cells. A vicious cycle has begun.

The process takes about 72 hours and the increased amount of fluid in the affected area of the brain is what is not able to be seen on the head CT. The swelling not only reflects injury, it can cause injury particularly by pressing the brain against the rigid bony walls of the skull. There is also a shift of the soft jelly-like brain through slits between the right and left side. This movement creates dangerously high pressure on the opposite side and is called "mid-line shift." Both sides of the brain are now affected, although the injury was initially limited to one side. There may be more of a change in level of consciousness and difficulties in thinking because of this involvement of both sides of the brain. The other major problem and one which could lead to death is shift of swollen parts of the brain pressing onto the brain stem. The brain stem controls the very process of breathing and maintenance of alertness. Thus, coma and death can result from swelling or brain edema following a stroke.

These effects of the injury to any part of the brain are the result of the size and site of the injury. These effects go beyond the specific area affected and extend to the entire life of the person. These effects are greatest at about 72 hours after injury. It is then that the effects are also greatest on the actions controlled by the brain and the patient looks his or her worst.

There are various methods available to deal with this increased edema. To remove the excess fluid, the water is pulled out of the brain by injecting a material into the blood vessels. One such material is called "mannitol." It is a large sugar molecule that increases the tendency of the blood to pull excess fluid from the tissue so long as the mannitol molecule remains intact. After a while, the mannitol is broken down into smaller sugars that no longer have the same effect. The effects of the mannitol don't last very long. Therefore, one needs to use it at the time when it is absolutely necessary to tide the person over until the swelling recedes of its own accord and the danger is lessened. The danger of death due to brain swelling early in the hospitalization is very great, particularly in those with hemorrhage.

What Can Cause Illness in Persons With Stroke?

A common cause of illness is the effects of the brain injury on the ability to swallow. People with difficulty in swallowing may have food pass not to the stomach but to the lungs. This can cause infection and possible death due to pneumonia. In order to maintain adequate nutrition, one bypasses the need for swallowing by use of a tube going to the stomach. This will be discussed in greater detail in Chapters 5 and 7. Still another problem that can cause serious difficulties with breathing and even death is clots forming in the legs when someone is in bed and unable to move. Clots in the deep veins of the legs may not be evident until there is a breaking off of a piece of a clot (embolism) that floats in the blood eventually reaching the lungs. The embolism lodges in a blood vessel in the lungs. There may be chest pain, difficulty breathing, and possible death. There are frequently no signs of the presence of these clots in the leg. It is therefore important to guard against their formation. One method in use is to prevent the stagnation of blood in the legs by the use of elastic stockings. Another possible intervention is to thin the blood to discourage clot formation by use of injectable drugs such as Heparin. Those who have had a hemorrhage are unable to use blood thinners such as Heparin. Another alternative is the use of a pump that is placed on the limbs to increase the return of fluid back to the heart to prevent stagnation.

Medically, what must be accomplished during this first week of hospitalization is to prevent illness that could lead to death due to infection and pulmonary embolism. Other medical challenges that may be faced are to prevent skin breakdown from lying in one spot in bed, to maintain adequate drainage of the bladder to prevent infection of the urinary tract, and to maintain movement of the bowels. Chapter 5 of this book goes into greater detail about the problems of illness in this early phase. During this first week, one can begin to look to what can be done to overcome the effects of the stroke. One can begin to see various degrees of recovery. One must avoid the use of drugs possibly affecting such recovery, and one must protect what has been injured. Therefore, if recovery occurs, there is a chance to regain the use of the foot, hand, or arm.

Where Does the Stroke Occur? What Part of the Brain Has Been Affected?

It can be confusing to realize that injury to one side of the brain affects the opposite side of the body. For example, injury to the left side of the brain may result in weakness or paralysis on the right side of the body. The brain as it lies in the skull is divided into two major parts; one connects with the spinal cord and extends to the point where the brain expands to fill the major part of the skull. The portion connecting the spinal cord to the larger part of the brain lies in the back of the head and is called the brain stem, like a stem on a plant. Injury to this small area can have very significant consequences because the centers controlling vital actions are very close together. A small hemorrhage, for example, can affect the coordinated control of all eye movements and cause blurred or double vision. Another small area of injury, for example, can affect control of swallowing including movements of the tongue and throat. The brain stem is also the only pathway of nerves carrying instructions for the arm or leg to move or carrying sensory information to the brain, such as a message that the shower water is too hot. A brain stem injury can block passage of this message. The person doesn't realize that the or she should pull the hand back and reduce the temperature.

The rest of the brain lies in the major part of the skull. Once again, it is divided into two major parts or hemispheres. The effect of the stroke is to interfere with function of the opposite side of the body, including control of the limbs as well as awareness of one's body in space and the feelings of touch and temperature. This includes vision because an injury to any portion of the nerve cells connecting the eye to the visual portion of the brain will generally affect the ability to see on the opposite side. Half of the field of vision is lost in each eye. Various parts of the brain are more commonly associated with control of limbs or sensation. The portion toward the front of the brain is associated with motor control; toward the middle and back with sensation; the furthest back with vision.

A "CT" scan of the head is an x-ray that may reveal the area of injury. MRI (Magnetic Resonance Imaging) may also be used as a diagnostic tool. The MRI shows up the difference between the areas of the brain that are injured from the rest by the different responses to a magnet. More recently, this same difference in response to the magnet can be used to outline blood vessels to determine blockage . This test is called MRA (Magnetic Resonance Arteriography). It is hoped that the use of this MRA can replace other tests to detect blocked blood vessels.

An injury to the left side of the brain in most persons affects the ability to use language, such as finding the right words. The problem is not merely expressing language by talking or writing, but also understanding what is written or said. One of the most devastating effects of stroke is this interference with human communication.

The injury from stroke results from something going wrong in the blood supply to the affected portion of the brain. The question of where the stroke occurred relates not only to the parts of the brain affected but the blood vessels which have been affected. Figure 1.1 illustrates the blood vessels that supply the brain. The brain stem has its blood supply from two blood vessels in the neck called the vertebral arteries named after how they run along the vertebra of the spine in the neck. These two arteries connect to form one artery that runs along the base of the brain stem and is called the basilar artery. These vessels cannot be easily reached from outside the body.

These arteries feed the major part of the brain on both sides of the neck, are, however, easily accessible to touch and also to be operated upon. They are called the carotid arteries, from the Greek meaning sleep. Pressure upon them could cause deep sleep. One of the questions to be answered is whether the stroke has been due to blockage of one of these major vessels in the neck. Surgery to clean out the ves-

Figure 2.1 Vascular Supply of the Brain

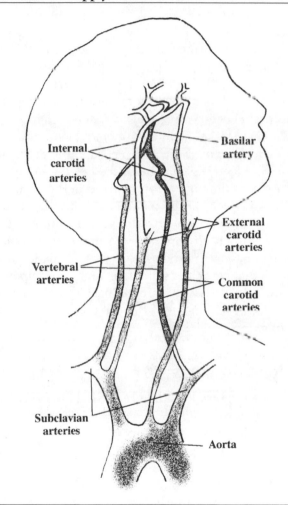

sel(s) (endarterectomy) could then be useful to prevent another stroke. There are several different techniques in use for improving the amount of blood going through these blood vessels. Some involve putting metal springs or plastic ducts into the artery to hold it open; others involve replacement of the affected blood vessel.

It is important to realize that the blood vessels going to the brain are part of a total system—the vascular system. The heart is the pump providing the blood carrying oxygen and nutrients to the brain as well as elsewhere. Any reduction in the strength of the heart will reduce the blood flow. The brain cells need a large amount of blood flow per minute to stay alive.

Atherosclerosis—hardening of the arteries—occurs in a patchy fashion and sometimes builds up in one blood vessel more than another. If there is a period of low blood pressure, from a heart attack or bleeding, the critical blood flow per minute to a portion of the brain with a cholesterol-choked vessel may not be enough to keep the brain cells alive. This is a stroke- an interruption of blood flow to the brain. Any reduction in blood pressure may make it difficult for the blood to get to the smaller blood vessels actually feeding the brain. Thus, when one looks for where the injury has occurred in the brain, it is necessary also to look not only at the blood vessels feeding that particular area but at the action of the heart. Although the injury may appear in either side of the brain, the problem lies in the overall blood supply. The damage that has occurred may be due to the inadequate ability of those vessels on that particular side of the brain to compensate for the lack of pressure. All the vessels are connected, but once again, with the development of hardening of the arteries, there may not be the ability to respond.

What Kind of Stroke is It?

The kind of stroke determines the effects and the consequent recovery. The question of what kind of a stroke has occurred and where it is can be answered by hearing the story of how rapidly it happened to that person and seeing the effects on the body of the person. This particular question is the one to be answered by that first head CT in the Emergency Department. There are two major kinds of stroke. One type is due to hemorrhage from a blood vessel rupturing (a bleed) and the other due to blockage of a blood vessel (a clot). The clot can come from the heart, or blockage can occur in the blood vessel wall itself.

A hemorrhage is what the doctor rules out with the first CT scan. Free blood is seen on the CT scan within minutes of a rupture. The swelling and resultant changes that mean there is a loss of blood supply or blockage may take as long as 72 hours to show up.

The first and most important question to answer is whether hemorrhage has occurred. The effects of hemorrhage may be deadly in the first few hours. Bleeding into the brain causes injury to brain cells by depriving them of their source of nutrients. The free blood itself can damage the ability of the cells to work properly. The blood will eventually be removed by scavenger cells and the damaged cells are also removed. The problems due to hemorrhage extend beyond the local damage. The presence of free blood can cause severe swelling of brain cells within the cramped space of the skull. This causes pressure on parts of the brain controlling breathing and consciousness. Bleeding and swelling within the brain cavity may cause coma, and the effects can lead to death within the first week.

Death of brain cells is also an effect when an artery in the brain is blocked. The brain cells starve to death and swell somewhat, but not as much as in a hemorrhage. Eventually, the dead cells are cleared away and a hole is formed. Even a small area of damage interferes with the function of the whole brain. All areas of the brain communicate with each other and help each other. When one "helper" dies, the rest of the brain slows down a little. This is called diaschisis. One of the opportunities for early recovery of function comes from reorganization of the rest of the brain to compensate for the lost brain cells.

How Severe is the Stroke?

The severity of the stroke can be measured in several ways. One way is to give a score of how much weakness there is in the affected limbs and how much feeling has been affected. Another scoring system is based on how well the patient can raise the limb itself. These are called impairment scales. A more meaningful measurement is to determine how much of regular daily activities the person with stroke can still carry out. These measurements are called disability or "activity" scales.

What Caused the Stroke?

This question can be answered several days after the stroke. If the stroke was caused by a hemorrhage, was it due to a break in an artery or vein in the brain? Arteriography must be done. A long, thin tube is inserted into an artery in the thigh then threaded up to the carotid arteries that supply the brain. A liquid that shows up on x-ray is injected through the tube and outlines the blood vessels so that good x-ray pictures can be taken. Alternatively, an MRA can also provide pictures of the blood supply. The arteriogram or "A"-gram still gives the best pictures.

If there was a blockage, it could have formed in place and is called a thrombosis, or it could have formed in the heart or carotid arteries and then floated into the brain, and called an embolism. Small, but dangerous clots form in the heart during the irregular heart beating rhythm called Atrial Fibrillation, that research suggests is a cause of stroke. The treatment will vary. Treatment with Coumadin®, a powerful blood thinner, has been found to reduce the likelihood of stroke. On the other hand, surgery is the best treatment if there is significant blockage (more than70 percent) in one or both of the carotid arteries. The blockage is caused by cholesterol deposits. These cholesterol deposits build up very slowly, but a crisis can occur if platelets start sticking to the lumpy, irregular areas of cholesterol plaques. Platelets help stop the bleeding in a cut by sticking together and forming a web over the opening in the blood vessel. If the blood vessel is not cut, then this sticking together can be quite dangerous. It can block the carotid artery, or a big clump of platelets can break free from the carotid artery wall and block another vessel in the brain. The sticking or clumping process is prevented using anti-platelet agents such as Aspirin, Ticlopidine (Ticlid) or Clopidogrel (Plavix). These drugs interfere with the clumping process and substantially reduce the risk of stroke from cholesterol deposits in the carotid arteries. A surgeon can peel these deposits away and leave clear vessels behind in a procedure named a "Carotid Endarterectomy."

Various tests are done to find the most likely source of blockage. An ultrasound study of the heart is done to find clots that could go to the brain. The name of this study is the 2-D echocardiogram and it is performed over the front of the chest. The EKG or electrocardiogram can tell whether there is a heart arrhythmia causing clots to form. Doppler ultrasound studies are done of the neck arteries to see how thick the cholesterol deposits might be.

How Can I Avoid Another Stroke?

The most common risk factor for stroke is high blood pressure (HBP). HBP may cause a stroke in two different ways. It damages the small blood vessels called arterioles (or little arteries) by thickening and weakening their walls. This can result in eventual blockage of the small blood vessels or rupture of the wall and hemorrhage. HBP also works on the larger vessels. There is increased likelihood of deposits of cholesterol in the walls of the blood vessels. The pounding of the blood when the pressure is high is thought to cause injury to the smooth inner wall of the artery, increasing the vulnerability to cholesterol deposits. The amount of fat in the blood affects the amount deposited on the arterial wall. Particularly important is the amount of fat in the diet. Cholesterol is an animal fat in foods such as butter, cheese and meat that is deposited in the arterial wall. This is discussed more fully in Chapter 6. Diabetes also affects the blood vessels throughout the body. Maintaining blood sugar within a normal range can reduce the likelihood of damage to blood vessels that can lead to blockage. All these problems tend to worsen with age.

Why Would a Young Person Have a Stroke?

The causes of stroke in younger persons are similar to those in older persons. High blood pressure, high cholesterol, and diabetes can be severe enough to cause strokes by hemorrhage or blockage. Another cause in both young and old is use of tobacco. Tobacco tends to increase clotting. Drugs such as cocaine are particularly dangerous in causing blockage by spasm of blood vessels or hemorrhage and can affect both young and old.

Sometimes there are abnormal portions of blood vessels in the brain such as an aneurysm (a ballooning or out-pouching in the wall of the blood vessel, usually located where one vessel branches into two or more vessels) or an arteriovenous-malformation (AVM- a tangle of abnormal, thin-walled blood vessels, all twisted and twined around each other, that shows up as a "blush" on an angiogram). Once an AVM is discovered, a neurosurgeon may decide to remove it because of the risk of bleeding. Similarly, an angiogram is performed to detect the suspected aneurysm. A neurosurgeon will find the aneurysm through angiogram and will place a little clip at the base of the bleeding aneurysm to stop the hemorrhage. HBP can also cause the aneurysm to bleed. The aneurysm is prone to bleeding since the walls of the pouch are very thin, and if the blood pressure rises, the pouch may pop and release blood into the brain. This is called a sub-arachnoid hemorrhage (SAH), and the person experiencing this "bleed" will complain of severe headache, maybe some neck stiffness, and become quite confused. The head CT will confirm the SAH.

In addition, there are abnormalities in the clotting of blood that can run in families. If certain blood elements are absent, there is an increased likelihood of clotting. Blood-thinning drugs are used to counteract this type of problem. Recent research has identified an excess of the amino acid homocystine as relating to stroke. The treatment here is to use the vitamin folic acid. Fortunately this vitamin is present in many multivitamin capsules available without a prescription.

What Can Happen Next In Getting Back to Life Again?

As the tests results become available and you have some answers about what has happened, it is necessary to begin looking to the future and setting goals. Some people go on to the future without answers to their questions in the acute stage. There is always another chance.

By the end of the first few days after a stroke, the medical problems have probably been brought under control and a plan implemented to help prevent another stroke. Now there needs to be a plan for retraining so that you can get back to living on your own as soon as possible. What is the best way to determine what kind of retraining would be necessary?

The various options for rehabilitation depend on your needs and resources (See Figure 2.2 "Care Path for People with Stroke"). For some, generally about a tenth of all strokes, there has been little impairment and there is a caregiver such as a spouse or daughter or son available to look after the patient to the extent that one is unable to care for him/herself at first. The location of rehabilitation for that person would be home. One can get whatever retraining is necessary either in the home or at an outpatient facility. The choice of either one would depend on the need for and availability of accessible transportation.

For those who have greater degree of impairment, it may not be possible to be cared for at home; or there is no one available to serve as a caregiver. These patients can not go directly home. If that person's impairments are so severe that he or she can not learn how to care for him or herself or be cared for, then rehabilitation is not likely to be successful. Inpatient rehabilitation is likely to be successful in about two-thirds of these cases, if the person has sufficient memory

Figure 2.2

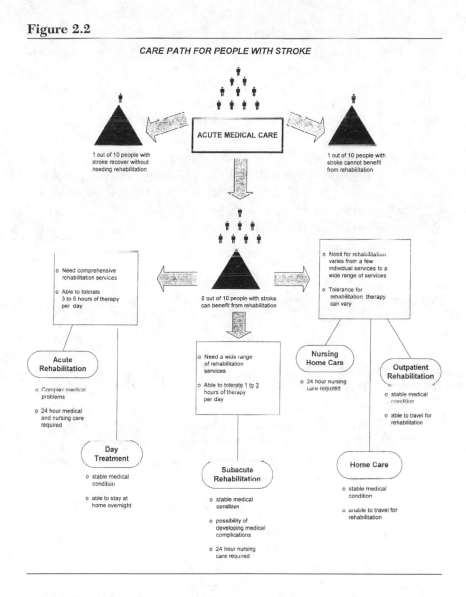

CARE PATH FOR PEOPLE WITH STROKE

ACUTE MEDICAL CARE

1 out of 10 people with stroke recover without needing rehabilitation

1 out of 10 people with stroke cannot benefit from rehabilitation

o Need comprehensive rehabilitation services

o Able to tolerate 3 to 5 hours of therapy per day

8 out of 10 people with stroke can benefit from rehabilitation

o Need for rehabilitation varies from a few individual services to a wide range of services

o Tolerance for rehabilitation therapy can vary

Acute Rehabilitation

n Complex medical problems

o 24 hour medical and nursing care required

o Need a wide range of rehabilitation services

o Able to tolerate 1 to 3 hours of therapy per day

Nursing Home Care

o 24 hour nursing care required

Outpatient Rehabilitation

o stable medical condition

o able to travel for rehabilitation

Day Treatment

o stable medical condition

o able to stay at home overnight

Subacute Rehabilitation

o stable medical condition

o possibility of developing medical complications

o 24 hour nursing care required

Home Care

o stable medical condition

o unable to travel for rehabilitation

and learning abilities to profit from the work of a team of professionals. They will work to teach him/her how to use what he or she has in
the way of function to use various assistive devices and to teach the
caregivers how to do their part. All these efforts are designed to reduce the amount of physical help needed from family or caregivers.

The intensity of the treatment provided will vary with the amount of medical and nursing supervision required along with the person's ability to participate in a more or less intensive program. Intensity is measured by the number and duration of services per day and per week. Ability to participate approximately three hours per day five days a week has been the general guideline for acceptance in the more intensive "acute rehab" facility. A person unable to benefit from or tolerate three hours per day of therapy may still benefit from a lower intensity of rehabilitation training provided in what is called a "sub-acute" facility. At times, the person may at first enter a sub-acute program and then be transferred to an acute rehab facility. The appropriate site for treatment follows guidelines developed by experts in the treatment of stroke.

Exercise 2.1 Asking Your Questions/Getting Answers (First Week)

This exercise can help you to review the questions you could have asked and help you define any other questions you might want to ask.

1. What were my concerns?

Check off those questions of concern for you that are now cleared up for you.

_____ 1. What happened when I had a stroke?
_____ 2. What is a stroke?
_____ 3. What happens next?
_____ 4. What can cause illness?
_____ 5. Where is the stroke ?
_____ 6. What kind of stroke was it?
_____ 7. How severe is the stroke?
_____ 8. What caused the stroke?
_____ 9. How can I prevent another stroke?
_____ 10. Why would a young person have a stroke?
_____ 11. What can happen next in getting back to life again?

Are there other questions that you want to ask? List them and try to get the answers.

_____

_____

_____

CHOOSING A REHABILITATION PROGRAM

- What do I need to know?
- What considerations will affect my choice of rehabilitation programs?
- Who can help me decide which rehabilitation program to choose?
- What kinds of rehabilitation programs are available, and how are they different?
- What kinds of rehabilitation professionals might I meet?
- Will I need more than one kind of stroke rehabilitation?
- How do I know what kind of rehabilitation program is right for me?

Selecting a medical rehabilitation program after you, a member of your family, or a close friend has had a stroke may be one of the most important and difficult medical decisions you ever make. See Appendix III for the Rehabilitation Program Checklist that will assist you in making this decision. The goal of this section is to answer your questions about how to select a rehabilitation program. You can check off on the front page of this section some of the questions you need to ask. At the end of this section you can once again check off the questions you have had answered, and identify any other questions you may still need to ask. (See "Life Outside Academe" in Chapter 11 for a graphic and poignant description of the trials and tribulations of having to make a rehab choice under duress.)

The more you understand about your medical condition and the kinds of rehabilitation programs that are available, the more involved you can be in making decisions about your stroke rehabilitation. Many of us think of medical rehabilitation in the same way we think of other medical treatment: If you have a broken leg, you get it set, let it heal in a cast for six weeks, and are then ready to walk again. This is not the case with medical rehabilitation. There is no magic pill or medical procedure that can help a paralyzed person suddenly walk again. Rehabilitation requires much patience, motivation, hard work, and time. Therefore, after a stroke, you must put aside notions of medical "cures" and think in terms of *relearning old skills*, such as how to walk and talk, and *learning new skills* in order to resume life despite the stroke. Your questions about choosing a medical rehabilitation program will be answered in the next section of this chapter. The next step is to understand the choices you will have in selecting a rehabilitation program.

Because of the rapidly growing cost of health care, many health insurance companies now control both the kind and amount of medical care that their policyholders may use. (See Chapter 3 for an up-to-date discussion of health insurance and coverage for medical rehabilitation). As a result, people today have fewer choices about their medical care than they had in the past. Nevertheless, the more you understand about your medical needs, your insurance coverage, and the treatment options available to you, the more prepared you will be to discuss rehabilitation options with your family, your doctor, and your **case manager**, as well as the person at your health plan who must approve your rehabilitation treatment (that is, the **gatekeeper**).

What Do I Need to Know?

To evaluate your options for rehabilitation, you need to know what kinds of programs are available and the type of rehabilitation coverage that your medical insurance provides. The next section of this guide, "About Rehabilitation Programs," provides a detailed description of rehabilitation programs and explains how they differ from one another. The following section, "Health Insurance and Rehabilitation," describes different kinds of health insurance plans and explains their coverage of rehabilitation services.

What Considerations Will Affect My Choice of Rehabilitation Programs?

The decision about which type of rehabilitation program to select depends on several things: the intensity of service needed (based on your level of impairment), your overall physical condition, and your insurance coverage. There are many different kinds of rehabilitation for people with stroke. The kind of rehabilitation services you receive will depend on several things:

- the severity of your impairment;
- the stability of your medical condition (that is, whether you are at risk for developing complications or having another stroke);

- your overall health and endurance, including your age and any chronic health problems you may have;
- the type of insurance coverage you have; and
- the availability of rehabilitation programs in your area.

Who Can Help Me Decide?

In addition to your doctor, a **medical social worker** at the acute-care hospital will be able to help you decide where to go for rehabilitation. He or she can also help you understand the specific features of your insurance coverage or Medicare entitlements, including the rehabilitation choices available to you and any restrictions or exclusions existing under your health plan.

What Kinds of Rehabilitation Programs Are Available, and How Are They Different?

There are many kinds of rehabilitation programs for stroke. These programs differ from one another in terms of the type of rehabilitation services they provide, how often they are provided, and the physical setting where services are provided. The different types of rehabilitation programs available are described. Stroke rehabilitation programs differ from one another in three basic ways:

- the type of rehabilitation services that are offered;
- the intensity of rehabilitation services that are offered (that is, how many times a week each service is offered and how long it lasts); and
- the setting, or physical location, of the treatment.

Acute rehabilitation programs provide both medical care and a full range of rehabilitation services, including physical therapy (PT), occupational therapy (OT), speech-language pathology (SLP), vocational rehabilitation (VR), audiology, psychology, orthotics/prosthetics, rehabilitation engineering, social services, therapeutic recreation, and pastoral care. Acute rehabilitation facilities develop personalized rehabilitation programs of different intensity and services to meet each patient's needs. Doctors are in direct contact with their patients (usually on a daily basis, but no less than three times a week) to monitor their medical condition and to evaluate their rehabilitation progress. Patients also receive a high level of nursing care. Patients treated in acute rehabilitation programs have complex medical needs and are at risk of developing complications if their medical treatment is not continued. However, to participate in an acute rehabilitation program, patients must be able to tolerate three-to-five hours of rehabilitation services per day for a minimum of five days a week. Acute rehabilitation programs can be found in freestanding rehabilitation hospitals and in specialized rehabilitation units that are part of general acute-care hospitals.

Subacute rehabilitation programs provide daily nursing care and a fairly wide range of rehabilitation services, including PT, OT, and SLP. Subacute rehabilitation is less intensive and generally lasts longer than acute rehabilitation. A subacute rehabilitation program consists of daily nursing care, a treatment plan supervised by a rehabilitation doctor, and medical management by a primary-care physician. Scheduled contact between the patient and the rehabilitation doctor is less frequent than in acute rehabilitation programs, often only once every two weeks. Since July 1, 1998, when the the government's Balanced Budget Act of 1997 was implemented, therapy services in sub-acute and long-term care have been drastically cut back. Be sure to find out from the sub-acute unit or nursing home what the person with stroke can expect in the way of rehabilitation services. Subacute rehabilitation is appropriate for patients with significant level of disability, but are unable to tolerate the amount or intensity of rehabilitation services provided in acute rehabilitation programs. Patients treated in subacute rehabilitation settings are medically stable, but need continued medical treatment to avoid possible complications. They are usually older or more frail than acute rehabilitation patients. Even so, they must be able to tolerate one-to-three hours of rehabilitation services per day.

Subacute rehabilitation is offered in many settings, including:

- freestanding subacute rehabilitation facilities,
- subacute rehabilitation units that are part of general acute care hospitals,

- freestanding skilled nursing facilities,
- skilled nursing beds located in residential nursing homes. Medicare does not recognize this level of care and it is only available through managed-care companies.

Day treatment is similar to acute rehabilitation, except that patients do not stay overnight in the hospital. Day-treatment programs offer a wide range of rehabilitation services supervised by rehabilitation doctors. Such programs provide three-to-five hours of rehabilitation services per day. Nursing care and general medical care are also provided as needed. Patients treated in day-treatment programs can benefit from intensive rehabilitation, but are medically stable and do not require an intensive level of nursing care or constant monitoring by a doctor. Day-treatment patients generally live at home or in some other residential living environment and visit the day treatment program three-to-five days per week. They are seen by the rehabilitation physician one to two times per week. Day treatment programs can be found as independent programs, as part of rehabilitation hospitals, or at **comprehensive outpatient rehabilitation facilities** (CORFs).

People receiving **outpatient rehabilitation** services live at home and travel to an outpatient facility for treatment. Outpatient rehabilitation can include a full range of services delivered as a coordinated program of care, or only one or two individual services, such as PT or OT. Typically, patients receive outpatient services two-to-three days per week. They see their rehabilitation physician one to two times per week. People receiving outpatient rehabilitation are medically stable and able to live in their own homes without risk of developing complications. Outpatient services are often prescribed as continuing treatment following more intensive rehabilitation in an acute—or subacute—rehabilitation program. Outpatient rehabilitation services are provided in many different settings, such as doctors' offices, hospital-based outpatient departments, hospital-owned outpatient centers that are located away from the hospital, and outpatient centers not associated with hospitals.

Home-care services allow patients to receive rehabilitation treatment in their own home. Rehabilitation professionals, such as nurses, PTs, or OTs, travel to the patient's home to provide rehabilitation services as often as their doctor has prescribed, usually one to three times per week for each type of rehab therapist. Home care is often ordered for patients who are able to live at home, but who are not able to travel to an outpatient facility because of their health, because they live too far away, or because they cannot easily get in or out their home due to disability.

Some, but not all, **nursing homes** provide rehabilitation services for their residents. However, the kinds of rehabilitation services offered and the intensity of the rehabilitation treatment can be very different from one nursing home to another. In general, nursing homes provide rehabilitation treatment two to three days a week. Treatment can be a single rehabilitation service, such as PT, or a coordinated program of care consisting of several different services, such as PT, OT, and SLP. Nursing homes, or **long-term care facilities**, are appropriate for patients who need continuous nursing care and cannot be cared for safely at home or in a residential living environment. Nursing home patients are medically stable, but they may have special needs that require nurses to be available 24 hours a day. It is important to understand two things about rehabilitation in nursing homes: first, not all nursing homes provide rehabilitation services; and second, nursing homes that offer rehabilitation are not all alike. Be sure to ask for specific details about the kinds of rehabilitation services offered, how often they are provided, and whether rehabilitation treatment is supervised by a rehabilitation doctor or another rehabilitation professional.

What Kinds of Rehabilitation Professionals Do I Need?

In the course of rehabilitation, you will most likely work with several different professionals. They make up your "rehabilitation team." The members of your team will vary, depending on your specific medical and rehabilitation needs, the type of rehabilitation program you are in and your insurance coverage.

- The rehabilitation doctor often leads the team and is responsible for medical decisions about your program of care. Stroke rehabilitation physicians are usually either neurologists or physiatrists, (specialists in physical medicine and rehabilitation) who have been trained to assess your problems from the stroke, monitor your health, and treat the medical complications.

- The rehabilitation nurse (CRRN) works with other rehabilitation professionals to personalize your plan of care. He or she assists you with activities of daily living and helps make your rehabilitation part of your daily routine. The rehabilitation nurse also teaches you and your family about your medication and how to prevent another stroke.

- The physical therapist (PT) evaluates your control of movement and your ability to function. He or she will have you perform specific tests to assess your strength, mobility and range of motion. Then the physical therapist designs a treatment plan to restore and maximize your movement and function based on the results of those tests. If you have difficulty walking or getting in and out of bed, then you need physical therapy.

- The occupational therapist (OT) teaches you skills and adaptation needed to increase your independence, productivity, and satisfaction at home, in the workplace and the community. Occupational therapies focus on preventing, reducing, and/or adjusting to your disabilities so you can perform a wide range of activities from bathing to managing personal finances. If your arm is clumsy or weak and you have difficulty bathing, dressing, or fixing some food, occupational therapy can be helpful to you.

- The speech and language pathologist (SLP) works to enhance your communication skills. This may involve helping you to improve your voice, speech, language, or conversational skills or teaching you how to use gestures, computers, or other devices to communicate. The SLP can also help you to adapt to difficulties with swallowing or eating, as well as impairments of your memory, problem solving skills and organization of your thinking.

- The therapeutic recreation (TR) specialist helps you to evaluate your leisure needs abilities and interests. Then the TR works with you to develop a treatment program. Therapeutic recreation activities take place in both the rehabilitation facility and the community and are designed to help you regain as much independence as possible by practicing your leisure time activities.

- The vocational rehabilitation specialist helps you to determine your job-related strengths, provides guidance for employment or education planning, and coordinates referral to community-based vocational rehabilitation services when appropriate. He or she might also offer training in how to look for a job and may consult with specific employers to encourage hiring and discuss necessary workplace modifications.

- The clinical psychologist helps you understand and adjust to your disability. The psychologist may provide training in different kinds of coping skills, such as stress management, pain control, or biofeedback, and may offer individual, family, or group counseling.

- Your medical social worker or case manager works with you, your family, and community agencies to make arrangements for a variety of support services. He or she can provide needed information, make referrals to community agencies, arrange for continuing care and provide counseling for individuals, couples, families, or groups. The case manager or medical social worker can help with the transitions to the community. The case manager also makes sure that all aspects of your treatment comply with the rules of your insurance coverage.

In addition to the members of the rehabilitation team described above, there are a number of other medical professionals whom you may encounter, depending on your needs. The audiologist uses advanced equipment to evaluate and diagnose hearing problems. He or she will make recommendations about the need for hearing aids or other assistive devices. The clinical pharmacist supplies medications prescribed by your doctor and is available to discuss your medications with you and your family. The neuropsychologist evaluates how an injury to the brain caused by the stroke affects behavior. He or she may give written or oral tests to assess cognitive abilities such as memory. The prosthetist/orthotist fabricates, fits and repairs artificial limbs and orthopedic braces. The registered dietitian develops a dietary plan to meet your personal nutritional needs and takes into account your food preferences, physical abilities and any dietary recommendations from your doctor. The rehabilitation engineer helps to select, modify and design assistive equipment for mobility, communication, work, recreation, and therapy. The respiratory therapist uses diagnostic equipment to assess your breathing and can help design a program to fit your individual needs.

Will I Need More Than One Kind of Stroke Rehabilitation?

During the course of your stroke rehabilitation, you may receive care in more than one program or setting. As your medical condition and rehabilitation needs change, you may be moved to a different program or treatment setting. This practice of moving patients between treatment programs and settings is known as a transfer between levels of care, and it ensures that you receive the correct kind and amount of rehabilitation throughout the entire course of treatment.

How Do I Know What Kind of Rehabilitation Program is Right for Me?

In addition to your doctor, your medical social worker and your case manager at the acute-care hospital will be able to help you decide where to go for rehabilitation. He or she can also help you understand the specific features of your insurance coverage or Medicare or Medicaid entitlements, including the rehabilitation choices available to you and any restrictions or exclusions exiting under your present plan.

Use information on rehabilitation programs located in Appendix B to help you evaluate and discuss your rehabilitation options with your family, your doctor, your medical social workers, and your case manager. The information on your health insurance coverage in the next chaper can help you to match your coverage with your needs.

Exercise 2.2 Asking Your Questions

This exercise can help you to review the questions you could have asked and help you define any other questions you might want to ask.

_____ 1. What do I need to know?
_____ 2. What considerations will affect my choice of rehabilitation programs?
_____ 3. Who can help me decide which rehabilitation program to choose?
_____ 4. What kinds of rehabilitation programs are available and how Ware they different?
_____ 5. What kinds of rehabilitation professionals might I need?
_____ 6. Will I need more than one kind of stroke rehabilitation?

_____ 7. How do I know what kind of rehabilitation program is right for me?

Are there any other questions you want to ask? List them below and try to get the answers.

_____

_____

_____

RETRAINING PHASE

- What does rehabilitation do?
- How is rehabilitation done?
- Will I get back to normal?
- How much recovery can I expect?
- Which functions will come back?
- How long will recovery take?
- What does therapy do for me?
- How can I prevent another stroke?
- How can I stay healthy?
- Can pain be a result of stroke?
- What kind of support will I need?

The goal of this section is to answer your questions now that it has been a week or so since the stroke has occurred. Your medical status is ideally more stable now. During the next few weeks, you will be getting treatment to help you to live at home. The goal of this section is to answer your questions about the stroke, about what recovery you can expect, and how to get back to living your life even if you do not have full recovery. You can check off on the front page of this section some of the questions you feel the need to ask. By the end of this sub-chapter, you should be able to understand how recovery happens, in what general order, and how long it might take. Finally, you will have another chance to check off the questions you had answered to your satisfaction and identify any other questions you may still have.

Besides the effects of the stroke on your body and the recovery you might experience, there are also questions about the effects of your stroke on your life. You should be able to understand how you can use what ability you have. Your abilities will let you do what you need to do.

Your goal is to be able to carry on with your life, get out of the hospital, and get home again. Some of the same questions you asked earlier may now be easier to answer. You may still be concerned about what caused the stroke. You should begin to ask about what you can do to prevent another stroke. The major concern for most patients is: what recovery can you expect and how can you get back to living your life?

What Does Rehabilitation Do?

Rehabilitation aims to do three things. The first is to protect what you haven't lost so that there will be no worsening of your situation. For example, one problem that you might experience on occasion is pain in an affected shoulder and hand. That pain can make it harder for you to move the arm and even make it stiffer. The stiffness can actually contribute to even more pain. It is helpful to keep the arm from getting stiff by moving it through the range of motion daily, even if someone else has to move it. The aim here is to maintain the arm so that, if motor control improves, there will be a non-stiff useful arm. The first aim of rehabilitation is to protect what you have.

The second goal of rehabilitation is to teach you ways of getting on with your life even if you still have trouble moving your arm or leg. There are many ways to get around. Walking is a great way, but it is not the only way. Catching a cab or using the elevator is part of a total system for getting around. That system is termed "mobility." Rehabilitation will teach you the different ways of getting around, how to use what you have and how to use helpful devices such as canes or wheelchairs. In addition, whoever is available to help you will be trained in your "mobility" needs.

The third goal of rehabilitation is to teach you ways of problem solving as times change and/or your body changes. There will always be new challenges and problems to solve. Rehabilitation will teach you to think about different ways of doing things. The question you must ask is: If one way does not work to accomplish what I want to do, what are other ways to reach the same goal?

How is Rehabilitation Done?

Rehabilitation is commonly carried out by a team of professionals working with the different problems you may have. The composition of the team may vary somewhat. The members of the team are described in detail in section 2 of this chapter. The rehabilitation hospital provides medical care, but the main focus is therapy to help the person with stroke and the caregiver learn how to improve enough to return home. An important rehabilitation principle is the importance of the patient, caregiver, and professionals working together as a team.

After a short assessment by the various team members, there will be a team meeting to develop a plan that includes the patient's probable discharge date, equipment needs, caregiver training, and need for further therapy after discharge. Team goals are set in areas that would particularly affect the ability of the person to go home. These are short-term goals such as getting on and off the toilet, bladder control, and getting up and down steps. Coordination between the team members' expertise and the patient's needs is a focus of the team meeting. There is review and revision of this plan during a weekly meeting while the patient is undergoing in-patient rehabilitation.

Will I Get Back to Normal?

Will I get my physical strength and my speech back? How about my mental capacities? Will I ever be back to the way I was before? The goal of most folks with a disability is to be the way they were before. It is unlikely that the person will be exactly as before. Because of the stroke, brain cells have died. Full recovery is unlikely. Yet the brain will recover to a considerable degree. Repeat brain CTs may still show an area of injury, even though the person may be walking and talking quite normally. Some brain cells are gone, yet the stroke's effects have almost disappeared. How this amazing recovery happens is not clear. However, recovery of many abilities does occur. One explanation involves cells that are near the stroke area initially stunned or disturbed during the first several days following the "brain attack." The nearby brain cells quickly regain their normal activity. In addition, the completely uninjured areas of the brain begin to take over the functions of the injured parts. The intact brain cells begin to develop new connections.

What Recovery Can I Expect?

In most cases there will be improvement after the stroke. How much and how fast improvement occurs varies with each person. As one might expect, it will differ depending on the extent of damage. The amount of swelling can vary with the amount of injury. The more injury, the more swelling; the more swelling, the more problems there are. There are also medications that can possibly interfere with early recovery. Which medications to avoid is not entirely clear. One group of medications to avoid are narcotics and those related to Valium. It is generally wise not to use any medications that act on the brain unless absolutely necessary.

The more improvement seen early, the more likely it is that lots of further improvement will occur later. The rate of improvement will vary not only with the amount of damage. Improvement tends to follow a particular pattern. The tendency is for the most improvement to occur in those parts of the body controlled by both sides of the brain. For example, slurred speech (dysarthria) will tend to recovery very nicely because both sides of the brain work on the lips and tongue muscles for producing speech. Another skill tending to return early is the ability to sit upright and maintain balance. The legs will return to strength at the hip and thigh sooner than at the ankle or foot. The body part least likely to improve is the arm, particularly the hand. Most often the shoulder and the elbow will show improvement before the hand. The hand is controlled almost entirely by the opposite side of the brain. It is therefore very sensitive to the effect of a brain injury. The hand, known for its "dexterity," is also the part of the body that performs some of the most delicate abilities, such as the ability to thread a needle, and thus it needs large numbers of uninjured neurons to do the work. The leg muscles are larger, and there are fewer neurons necessary per muscle to do the job. Even if there are only a few brain-leg neurons left, they can control the leg enough to be able to walk, but perhaps not enough to jump or dance.

The pattern of recovery is affected by still another factor that reflects the evolution of the brain. The oldest part of the brain is related to balance and maintenance of balance. Balance recovers early. The muscles which "oppose gravity" also recover early. In the legs, the muscles that work against the tendency to fall are those causing the leg to remain straight (extended) at the hip and the knee. This is very helpful to persons with stroke since they will be able to stand if there is hip extension and knee extension, and they don't fall by losing their balance. Walking requires bending (flexion) of the leg at the knee and hip and generally occurs later than standing. The anti-gravity position of the arms with bent elbows is less helpful. The tendency of the weak arm to go into flexion at the elbow and fingers is a kind of recovery. If the arm is not stretched regularly, however, it can get stuck in this position, called flexion contracture. To avoid contractures, therefore, you are encouraged to provide passive range of motion to your fingers and wrist to keep your involved hand flexible.

What Function Will Come Back?

There are different levels at which we analyze the way the body works. The first level is that of the muscles themselves. When muscle actions are tested, it is usually in relation to control of a joint. In order to flex the elbow, it is necessary for the opposing muscle to relax. The coordination of flexion of the one and relaxation of the other is necessary. After a stroke, even when the muscle strength is regained, the coordination may be lost. It is important to understand that the muscles themselves are not weakened by the stroke, nor are the nerves going directly to those muscles. The injury is in the brain where coordinating of the contractions and relaxations of muscles takes place. Ultimately, multiple actions are coordinated into a complex activity, such as dressing. The functional movement at a joint is "impaired" by a stroke. Ultimately, what is important is how the impairment changes or interferes with the ability to dress, talk, or walk.

As noted before, the term "disability" is used to describe the effects of such impairments on your activities of daily living. The lack of coordination or weakness at the elbow joint may make it difficult to dress. The lack of coordination or weakness in particular actions of the legs may make it difficult to walk. These disabilities may be overcome, even if the impairments remain. You can learn to dress yourself by learning new ways of doing it with only one hand. You can learn to get around by learning how to use a wheelchair rather than walk, or to use a cane and brace to enable you to walk safely even, if not exactly the way you did before. The disability in "getting around" can be solved even if the leg impairment remains. An important part of rehabilitation is to learn to accomplish the things that count in your life, even if you need to do it in a different way than before.

How Long Will Recovery Take?

Recovery goes on for weeks and months,. There is no absolute limit to recovery, although most recovery tends to occur during the first few months. After this time, recovery tends to slow and "max out" after a year. An example of the pattern of recovery and the time frame in which it can occur is the case of a 58 year-old woman who hand a hemorrhage in the right side of her brain and required removal of the blood clot. She had had a sudden onset of weakness and numbness over the entire left side of her body. There was initially no movement at the shoulder, elbow, or wrist. There was some hip and knee extension, but no movement at her ankle. Within two months, she had more control of her hip with some at the knee, but still none at the ankle. She could move at the shoulder with some pain, but not well at the wrist. Within four months, she was moving her wrist and hand. Within six months, she was able both to use her hand to dress herself and to walk with a brace and a cane. It was not until seven months after her injury that she could now begin to control her ankle. The next month, she was using her arm in carrying out her household activities and experienced somewhat better control at the ankle. During the time that these actions were not available at the ankle and at the hand, she did not merely wait for them to return. She continued to get around, even if using a brace. She continued to work at finding new ways to dress herself even when the hand did not yet work that well.

Another patient had a stroke affecting his right side and his language and thinking. He found the problems using his right hand interfered with his ability to do certain activities during a lecture that were a necessary part of his job as a teacher. He was at first unable to understand and write what he wanted to do. He found a way to type what he wanted to say. At first he could not write more than a word at a time. Gradually, he begin to write sentences and then paragraphs. Each month and each year he was able to do more. He did not give up and he found that significant improvements continued to occur even several years later. If you don't use it, you lose it. If you do use it, you will continue to gain.

The person with stroke will get some muscle control back in most instances, but the important issue is being able to do things for oneself. Movement of a muscle that had not previously moved is a sign of "recovery." But the question one asks is, "Will I be able to do things I need to do, now that my muscle can move?" The answer to that question comes from a different level of understanding of the concept of "recovery."

When most people think of recovery, they mean doing what they could do before the stroke. Doctors tend to think of recovery beginning from the moment after the stroke. One man who had problems affecting all four extremities due to an injury, ended up with just a limp on one side. To anyone who saw him it would seem he had made an extraordinary recovery. However, he was disappointed because he compared himself to the way he was before his stroke.

It is natural to want to be without any problems. However, some brain cells have been lost. It is rare to see recovery of "100%." Even if there is eventual substantial return, it would be foolhardy to just wait for that to happen and not try to learn to care for yourself and be able to get around as soon as possible. You don't have to give up on living and doing what is important just because you still have trouble moving your arm or leg. "Recovery" can mean getting back to life again.

Terrible things happen to many people. If you are still alive, you must and can learn to carry on. NRH's credo is a timely reminder to us all: "*adding life to years* with service, compassion, and pride." It is not just a matter of the passage of time. Some people have been told that recovery will go on for the first three months and think that will happen regardless of what they do, that the brain will just do the job. This is not the way it works.

What Does Therapy Do for Me?

There is some confusion about rehabilitation. What makes a difference in your actual performance? How does the therapist contribute to it? Often the assumption is that the therapist makes you better. It is more useful to consider the therapist as a coach who helps you to realize your own potential. The therapist can teach you exercises and other activities to maintain range of motion, to prevent stiffness and injury to the affected limbs, and how to position them to prevent future problems. In addition, therapists can help you choose an appropriate cane, walker, or brace. He or she can teach you to learn how to use these things to get around and proceed with life at home. The third aspect is that therapists can enable you to learn various strategies about walking, dressing, going to the bathroom, and talking. The therapist can also help you learn to discover new strategies for yourself after therapy has stopped.

What Can I Do to Avoid Another Stroke?

The first thing that you can do for yourself is to stop smoking. This is a well known cause of stroke, cancer and heart attack. Additionally, there are several causes for blood clots forming in the heart and can then travel to the brain, such as too much alcohol, atrial fibrillation, and artificial heart valves. There are drugs called "blood thinners" that can cause the blood to be less likely to form clots. Your job would be to take those drugs. Anti-platelet drugs such as aspirin, Ticlopidine, and Plavix are one group. Another group of drugs actually slows down the clotting mechanism. Other treatments reduce the possibility of hemorrhage and the wear and tear on blood vessels caused by hypertension. Successful treatment is very much in your hands. Not only taking medication, but learning how to modify your diet and learning stress management can help in controlling your blood pressure. This is discussed in greater detail in Chapter 6 of where there are plans to deal with the "risk factors" causing stroke

What Can I Do to Stay Healthy in General?

The problem causing stroke is not just in the blood vessels of the brain. The blood vessels going to the brain are similar to the ones going to the heart, the arms, and the legs. Poor blood supply to the heart can cause heart attack and death from pump failure or abnormal heart rhythm. Treatment to lower the clogging by cholesterol in these arteries has been shown to be very helpful. Persons with diabetes are particularly likely to have problems with blood vessels. It has recently been shown that careful treatment of persons with diabetes can lessen vascular complications such as stroke. Diabetic atherosclerosis is the main cause of amputation of the legs. These aspects are also discussed more fully in Chapter 6.

Can Pain Be a Result of Stroke?

Pain can occur after a stroke. There are two kinds of pain. One type is generally limited to the affected body part, for example, pain occurring in the shoulder and/or in the hand. This pain can be severe, and there are a number of ways to treat it. One way to prevent pain from occurring is to be sure that people are very careful to not pull on the weakened arm while moving in bed or while transferring. The pain might not show up until after the first few weeks. Another type of pain may show up even later. It is called "central post-stroke pain." It shows up on the affected side of the body. This pain, sometimes very severe, can also be treated. There are methods to reduce the effect of the pain. It is important to be aware that this sort of pain can occur. Many people, including some physicians, may not connect this pain with the stroke because the time elapsed may be several weeks or months after the stroke. It is treatable. Both types of pain are discussed more fully in Chapter 5.

What Kind of Help Will I Need After I Leave the Hospital?

The amount of help you need upon discharge from the hospital can be a moderate amount of physical assistance or just supervision. The amount of physical assistance needed can also vary from someone just guiding you or actually doing some lifting. The amount of lifting that any caregiver can do on a regular day-to-day basis is limited. We try to get the stroke survivor to the point where he or she does at least 75% of his own lifting before discharge home.

The purpose of rehabilitation is to enable you to carry on in your home with the least amount of support. Even after you go home from the hospital, you can get therapy in your home or at an outpatient rehabilitation center. The therapy that will help you to continue to increase your ability to care for yourself. The support available after you go home depends on many factors. Who is available to help care for you if you can't take care of yourself entirley? Are there family members? Are other resources available? Can you afford to hire someone? The first task is to determine your needs and then the resources available. The rehabilitation team will work with your caregivers so that you will be cared for safely. This training is an important part of rehabilitation.

There is only a limited amount of support available from Medicaid, Medicare, or insurance for managing in your home. The laws do change, and there is much variation to what is available between states and regions of the country. Medicare, a Federal health program for elderly persons, can provide support for medical costs but does not ordinarily provide support for medicines or round-the-clock care. It may provide for a home health aide to come in several times a week for a short time per day. This issue is addressed more fully in Chapter 3.

One important issue is whether you know how to get the help you need. If you contract with helpers, you need to learn how to have people help you without taking away your independence. It is a matter of control. Who is in charge? Do you make the decisions? Quality of life consists of being able to manage your own life, deal with your own problems, and learn what works best for you. Caregivers should not merely give care but enable the person to care for him or herself.

Exercise 2.3 Asking Your Questions/Getting Answers

This exercise can help you to review the questions you might have asked, and to check off those that you have had answered to your satisfaction. You can also now define any other question you may want to ask.

_____ 1. What does rehabilitation do?
_____ 2. How is rehabilitation done?
_____ 3. Will I get back to normal?
_____ 4. What recovery can I expect?
_____ 5. Which function will come back?
_____ 6. How long will recovery take?
_____ 7. What does therapy do for me?
_____ 8. How can I prevent another stroke?
_____ 9. How can I stay health?
_____ 10. Can pain be a result of stroke?
_____ 11. What kind of support do I need?

Are there other questions that you now want to ask? List them below and try to get the answers.

_____
_____
_____
_____

COMMUNITY LIVING

- When will I be independent?
- What recovery can I expect?
- How can we deal with change in our relationship?
- What about sex?
- How to deal with feelings about myself, about self-image?
- Why do I cry so much?
- How can I get around?
- Can I get back to work?
- How can I prevent another stroke?
- Are there restrictions about my use of alcohol?

By this phase, generally about four weeks after the stroke, you can take care of many of your basic needs. You are now at home, but still experiencing the effects of your stroke. The goals are different. Your goals are no longer limited to getting in and out of bed or dealing with your basic bodily needs. "Activities of daily living" are much wider in scope. Shopping, as well as meal preparation, and managing your money are examples of what you may want do to regain control of your life. Also important are those activities that give meaning to life - returning to your hobbies and/or to your work and getting back to your social, family, and religious life. Many stroke survivors are finding that they still need help in getting around and are frustrated with their degree of dependence.

New questions are coming up as you spend time at home again. You can check off on the front page of this section some of the questions you want to ask. One question remains about the recovery you can continue to expect. You may still be bothered by what you can do to keep from having another stroke. The questions remain, but the answers may change. At the end of this section, you can once again check off the questions that you have had answered to your satisfaction and identify any other questions you may want to ask. Now that you have had much more experience, it is likely that your own new questions will be even more numerous and be much more specific to yourself.

When Will I Be Independent?

The concept of independence depends on your perspective. The word "independent" means different things to different people. Many consider getting around by driving themselves as most important. For some it means never needing any help from anyone. But there are very few of us who do not depend on others for at least some part of our lives. With many married couples, one may pay the bills or prepare most meals. Many adults help their elderly parents with groceries and laundry, although the parents live by themselves. Independence can be described as the ability to choose how you conduct your life. The aim of becoming more independent is to be able to make decisions and to control your own life. It may be necessary to have help in areas that did not in the past require assistance. There may be a need for learning new ways of getting things done, including telling others how to do it. Dependence is not the need for assistance, but the loss of choice over how you are assisted. The major rehabilitation questions then is, "how actively can I *participate* in society?"

By now you have learned how to use some compensatory strategies to carry out your basic life activities. What worked for you in the hospital may no longer work in the community setting. During this period of your recovery, you may want to take an even more active role in defining some of your difficulties and goals. Everyone tends to have similar plans while in the hospital. Different people have different needs back at home and in their own communities. You are now at home and the problems you have are specific to your own situation. That situation will vary mainly with the type of housing you have and the availability of caregivers.

If you are independent in a wheelchair but cannot walk, you still can return to your ranch-style house or third-floor apartment with an elevator. If your home is two stories and the only bathroom and bedroom are upstairs, many more problems will need to be solved. You may need a bedside commode or someone to assist you up the stairs. Many stroke survivors worry that they will be a "burden" on their families. There are several reasons why this is an unfair description to accept. In most cases, the family is so happy to have their loved one alive and at home, even if disabled, that they don't mind helping you. Also, the need for assistance may be temporary, especially if you are doing the exercises recommended by the therapists. Finally, your family can see you becoming progressively more independent, and they will be happy and proud of themselves that they supported you in your time of need. Most likely, you would do the same for them if the "shoe were on the other foot."

You may continue to receive various types of therapy. This is another opportunity to participate actively in making plans for your own recovery. The therapist will bring expertise and you will bring knowledge of your daily needs and problems to the planning process. You know what helped you make progress during in-patient therapy sessions. You have a good sense of what you can accomplish over time. You also know what works during the night and weekends, when no therapist is present. Share this knowledge with your therapists. Work together as partners to achieve greater independence.

One woman with stroke who had gone home with continued weakness of her arm and leg wrote a diary about her goals and what she discovered that worked for her.

> I wanted to do things I had done before my stroke. I decided I would pick a new task and try to do it. The first task I picked was making Christmas place mats. I didn't know how I would do it, but I started to work. It took me a whole day to make five where it usually took about one hour. I did get them done.
>
> Next day, I did something else I used to do. I took my cane and a gallon bucket and went out on my hillside and picked a gallon of blackberries. (I hooked the bucket to my cane until it was about half full, and then set it on the ground so it wouldn't topple over.) I didn't get any more scratches than usual. Did I ever enjoy them that night! Next day I gave some to a neighbor. I could share them again and that made me feel real good too.
>
> Well today I decided to try something difficult. I'm going to clean my oven today. It hasn't been cleaned since April and it was a mess. I sprayed it early with oven cleaner and let it set for a couple of hours. I figured I could get at the front but how would I clean the back? So I went looking for something to use. I decided a long handled toilet brush might work so with a bucket of water a rag and the brush I started to work. Got all I could with the rag then tried the brush. It just smeared stuff around so I put the rag over the brush and presto it worked. It took about six changes of water but now the oven really looks clean again. I think my next project will be to scrub the kitchen floor.
>
> I've learned something. Now if I don't try to do some of my old jobs, how will I know I can't do them again and whether I need to start learning a new way. The only thing that can stop me is failing to try. A new way can be devised for almost any job and I'm sure going to try to find it.

This case illustrates the point that she found out not only what might work, but also that there are many ways of doing things, of "participating in her prior activities with gusto and guts."

What Recovery Can I Expect?

The question asked in earlier phases can be asked again. One man who was able to get around on his own with a cane continues to have problems with a hand that goes into spasm. He still asks the question that he asked earlier. Now it has changed to reflect his experience. His concern now is whether he can continue to expect improvement even eight months after his stroke. "When does recovery stop? What hope is there for more recovery now that I reached a 'plateau?'" The word refers to when therapists note that progress has become too slow to continue regular therapy.

The rate of return of arm/leg control and of speech and language is the best measure of the return that might occur. If you have had some return, it is likely that you will have more. The earlier the return has occurred, the more likely there will be substantial return. Return of hand function is particularly problematic in persons with stroke. There may have been return of action in the leg, but not in the arm. The important issue is to protect potential future function by keeping the hand and arm flexible and to use it as much as possible. This will also help prevent chronic pain in the arm. Focus on the return of motor control can be counter-productive and frustrating without an attempt to use what one has at present.

Many have been told that return occurs in time over the first six months. The idea that there will be return merely by waiting doesn't work. The most significant recovery will generally occur in those people who do the most work. One such case was that of a 57-year-old woman who had a stroke with residual difficulty in control of her left hand. It was about eight months since her stroke. She was only then able to focus more directly that she needed to stretch and exercise and use that hand in order to regain more function again. She had not been able to work and had become depressed about the situation because her hand was still somewhat impaired. She believed she had been promised improvement in the hand over the first six to eight months. She expected that it would return completely to normal and that she didn't even need to work on helping the recovery process.

Unfortunately, there had not been much improvement. The problem now was that the hand was not back to normal and in addition, she experienced a sense of helplessness caused by waiting for recovery to happen. If she had worked to improve the hand function and to find new ways to fulfill her job responsibilities, there would have been a sense of accomplishment of overcoming obstacles.

The term recovery means different things depending on your approach to life. For some, it remains that they want to be just as they were before the stroke. For others, the stroke is accepted as a harsh reality and recovery means going on with life and making the best of what strength and willpower is available. One can take the initiative in finding new ways of carrying out one's daily activities. One person for example was able to carry on with her cooking with the use of some adaptive utensils and some minor changes to her kitchen. Another woman returned to being a good mother by using a logbook and some extra planning. Stroke recovery is only a problem for those who insist that they aren't normal until they are just as they were before the stroke. Normal is what you are right now, not what you were months ago or ten years ago.

It has been helpful for some to think about the difference between what you want to do and how you go about doing it. The "what" is the end, the goal; the "how" is the means, the tactics or strategies you use to get you there. On some level most people would like to do things the way they have always done them. They would like to regain that old, customary way. Sometimes that is possible. Unfortunately, one generally has to use alternative ways to accomplishing many of the things you want to do. The most obvious example is being able to write if the stroke affected your writing hand. Most people can learn to write using the other hand. Some can write with a typewriter or a personal computer. Recovery also means learning more precisely how your body reacts and becoming master of your body once again. In order to make a good transition to the new way of thinking, there is still another level of recovery that becomes even more important. That is the recovery of one's sense of self-esteem and a sense that you can run your own life.

One lady with stroke with left-sided weakness had considerable difficulty with arthritis as well as the stroke. Her weight had always been a problem but now caused her particular difficulty. She was unable to get herself from sitting to standing and get to the toilet or in and out of bed. She still was unable to get around until about eight months after her stroke when she began to make noticeable progress. For the first time, she did not need someone to help her life herself up. She was able to get up without any actual physical assistance. When she was asked about what worked, she said "I finally told myself to do that . . . I want to use the skills I have been taught . . . I remember what you said at the beginning that I have to take charge . . . I need now to take charge!"

Another woman who had been a writer had marked difficulty in balance interfering with transfers and walking for several years after her stroke. She had initially been in a nursing home but was able to get back to her own home when she learned how to transfer with less help. She was able to find a caregiver now that her level of assistance was more manageable. Over the months she gained further control over her body and learned to shift her weight to compensate for the problems in balance. Her breakthrough was not immediate, but gradual. Each step required attention and hard work. Part of her strength and perseverance came when she once again found an opportunity to write about what she was experiencing. She had worked out a way to use a tape recorder despite her weak left hand. With some modification of the keys she was once again able to dictate her ideas. It was this success that was supportive to her sense of well-being and that enabled her to keep up the effort necessary to progress in her other motor skills.

How Can We Deal With the Change in Our Relationship?

Getting along with your mate who is taking care of you can be more of a problem than before. Changes in the roles between spouses can be a major concern affecting all aspects of marital life. One such case was that of a 55-year-old man who had been a high-level manager in his work before experiencing a brain hemorrhage several years before. He had residual left-sided weakness and it interfered with his gait. Of greater significance was pain in his affected side that interfered with his ability to carry on with his life. He had been told that such pain was to be expected after a stroke. He had been depressed about the progress he had made because of the feeling of helplessness caused by the pain. His physicians's statement that such pain was to be ex-

pected did not provide him with any opportunity to deal with it effectively. He felt, therefore, that it was not something he could do
anything about. The pain became the focus of his life. It justified not
taking charge of other aspects of his life that he could perhaps do
something about. His wife was concerned about his depression and
lack of initiative. What troubled her most was his abdication of his role
in caring for the family finances. She had never been able to do so in
the past and was particularly frustrated about being forced to do so
now. There were several things that could have been done to remove
or at least lessen the effects of the pain on his life. He finally learned
to control the pain and not let the pain control him. When he finally
used these methods, he also began to take more initiative in other aspects of his life.

What About Sex?

The major issues in marital life are those relating to body image and
changes in role. These are not necessarily related to the degree of actual impairment, but to the effects of such impairments on the person
experiencing them. One major area in which this sense of loss trans-
lates into dysfunction is that of sexuality after stroke. There are several different kinds of concerns in relation to sex. Some ask whether
having sex can be dangerous, particularly to the male. The answers to
this question include the way intercourse is accomplished as well as
the time of day. Poor communication and lack of information can add
to the problems of resuming a satisfying sexual relationship. Many
wives of men with stroke were afraid of "injuring" their husbands.
These wives also felt that their husbands were "afraid" to take part in
sexual activity.

Each concern can aggravate the difficulty with sexuality. Failure to
communicate with the other is really the underlying problem. One
piece of information can help to deal with the fear. In counseling the
patient with hypertension, it is important to emphasize that the inci-
dent of cerebral hemorrhage is not necessarily related to activity during sexual intercourse. Hypertension tends to be more severe in the
morning. If it is of concern, the time of sexual intercourse could be
adjusted to make it safer. Furthermore, to reduce the degree of elevation in blood pressure during sex, the male with hypertension can sit
on a low, wide chair with his feet on the floor with his partner on top.

What are the other answers about what to do if sex is not going well? Medications can have an adverse effect on the sexual functioning of an individual, such as causing impotence or reducing sexual desire. Of particular concern are drugs to treat hypertension. Many of these drugs act on the system allowing erections and ejaculation. Medications can be changed so that they would be less likely to cause difficulty. Clinical depression after stroke has also been linked to problems with impotence and decreased libido after stroke. Treatment with appropriate medication may be helpful or sexual counseling may be of benefit to enhance awareness and lessen anxiety.

How to Deal with Feelings About Myself, About Self-Image?

One person with longstanding left-sided involvement described her problem.

> The ongoing presence of the impairment made me feel out of "synch." My self-image, past experience, and how I saw myself did not match what I called my "mirror image," what I saw in the mirror. My body image, my self-image, and my self-esteem, these nebulous concepts about myself, were no longer based on reality. They were based on the able-bodied person I had been, and they included a bias against disabled people. As a child, I had seen legless veterans from W.W.I begging on the streets when I would be going to the movies on Saturdays with friends. I had judged these men to be pitiful creatures. Becoming disabled did not eliminate this prejudice. I undoubtedly complicated my emotional recovery.
>
> Ads are designed to point out that it is bad to have a physical flaw. But now there does not seem to be any way to hide the flaw. I felt I was a false being. This thoroughly unnatural combination of pre-stroke image in post-stroke body made me uncomfortable in my own presence. This probably made other people uncomfortable with me as well. I never actually gave up hope of returning to my pre-stroke self. At last, I realized I would never "recover." It was one of the most liberating experiences I have every had, because at last I was in touch with my reality. No more wasting time chasing impossible dreams. I could focus on the present and no longer looked backward to what used to be "nor-

mal," but focused on my new normal of being a capable disabled lady. I was finally back in "synch." Being in synch provided energy for subsequent endeavors. I was comfortable in my own presence. I could make what I chose of life; I was filled with pride and dignity. I may not have as many options as I formerly did, but isn't the lesson of life learning to do the most you can at a particular time?"

Sometimes one needs to modify the goal as well as the means used to get there. It becomes necessary to go to another level of thinking about one's goal. The person with longstanding effects of her stroke has compatible with ongoing difficulties and to regain control of one's life by reordering one's goals as well as the means to accomplish those goals.

Why Do I Cry So Easily?

Many people, women and men, find themselves having frequent outbursts of tears called "lability." This is a normal response to the very unpleasant experience of the stroke. It is very frustrating and depressing, but in addition, the stroke frequently takes away the ability to mask or control your emotions. All people have quick flashes of anger, happiness, sadness, or joy when they see a beautiful baby, or hear some special music. We don't show all of these little emotional moments because we may keep them to ourselves. The stroke survivor may have lost the ability to hide these emotional moments, and then he or she gets embarrassed at showing himself, and the person gets even more emotional. This problem usually comes back under some control, although it is always ok to show a little emotion. A person with stroke once described this condition as "I'm depressed because I'm crying; I'm not crying because I'm depressed."

How Do I Get Back to Getting Around? How About Driving?

Many people return to driving after stroke. Certain issues may develop after a stroke which could affect your ability to drive safely. They include:

- decreased movement of an arm or leg,
- difficulty understanding or reading traffic signs,
- loss of vision on one side of the body,
- inattention to affected side (neglect),
- difficulty adjusting to rapid stimuli and making judgments in busy traffic,
- possibly having had a seizure.

Most states require a person who experiences a neurological injury or illness serious enough to require hospitalziation to report this fact to the motor vehicle administration before returning to driving. There is a section on the medical evaluation form that your doctor must complete about whether your medical condition may affect your safety when driving. If this form contains information that raises questions about a person's ability to drive safely, the local motor vehicle authorities may call the individual in for an interview or require additional testing. Most auto insurance policies require that a person who experiences an illness or injury requiring hospitalization report that fact to the auto insurance carrier before returning to driving. If a person fails to do so, the insurance carrier can use this as grounds to refuse to cover the driver in the event of an accident. Driving rehabilitation is available at a number of rehab centers that can evaluate a person's safety while driving and provide on the role instruction to improve driving skills. There are generally several options available for transportation in the event that an individual is unable to use normal public transportation. Transportation for a variety of essential needs can be arranged through community, public, and/or voluntary organizations. For more specific information regarding the transportation services available in your area, you can contact any of the following agencies that exist in your community: the Transit Authority or the Council on Aging (See Appendix A for a host of post-stroke resources that you can access in your community).

Can I Get Back to Work?

If an older or disabled person's capabilities do not match the demands of the environment, the environment can be changed. Many environmental communication barriers are slowly disappearing, largely as a result of the Americans with Disabilities Act of 1990. In addition,

ADA prohibits employment discrimination against "qualified individual with disabilities." A person with a disability is defined as an individual who has a physical or mental impairment that substantially limits one or more of his or her major life activities. Persons who had a stroke would fit this definition. A "qualified" person is someone who can carry out the essential requirements of the job with reasonable accommodations. It is necessary to identify what your job really requires you to do. The next step is to figure out how, with reasonable accommodation, you can carry out that job. Employers cannot discriminate against individuals with disabilities in any employment practices or terms, conditions, and privileges of employment. This prohibition covers all aspects of the employment process, including the application and testing stages and all other aspects of the job. A vocational rehabilitation therapist is well versed in the ADA law and should be able to assist you in deciding whether employment might be a real possibility for you.

How Can I Prevent Another Stroke?

During the earlier phases of your life after stroke, you will have identified some of the risk factors over which you may have had some control. These include use of tobacco, the management of hypertension, the lessening of the build-up of plaques in the arteries due to high cholesterol. They also include lessening the likelihood of clots coming from the heart or other blood vessels by use of medication to reduce the tendency for clots to form. (See Chapter 6 for an extensive discussion regarding how to prevent another stroke.)

During the earlier phase of your recovery, you ideally would have learned the goals you are trying to achieve in order to reduce the likelihood of another stroke. For example, the goal for tobacco would be to stop smoking. The goal for hypertension may be to keep your blood pressure no higher than a certain number. Most folks try to keep the blood pressure below 140/85 but the specific numbers can vary with your age and other factors. A goal can be established between you and your physician relating to each of the areas covered by stroke prevention.

You may also have learned some of the things that you could do to achieve those goals. In many instances, medications can help. You would need to learn what those medications are, what they care called, and what dose and time to take them. You would also know what to watch for in the way of side-effects. You are now also able, in at least the case of blood sugar and blood pressure, to record your own progress. You and your physician can see for yourself whether you are meeting your goals. This process of "Making a Plan for Myself" is described in Chapter 4 of this book and is illustrated at the end of each of the problem areas that you can identify throughout the rest of the book.

In many instances, the medication cannot work alone. It is necessary for you to manage your diet to reach the goals. Diet in the case of diabetes means reduced carbohydrate load and smaller and more frequent meals. As in other instances, exercise coupled with diet enhances your control. In the case of the use of blood thinning drugs, you need to know which foods contain Vitamin "K" which works to counteract the effect of the drugs. Lowering your cholesterol in your blood requires you to lower the fat in your diet.

Now that you are on your own, the results depend on what you choose to do. You know your goal and you know what is recommended for you to achieve that goal. In some instances, you can even keep checking with yourself to see if you are achieving that goal. When you can's check with yourself, at least at present, you can ask your doctor to check it out for you. You need to set up a plan with your doctor about when to sound an alarm. When is the blood pressure so high or so low that action is required? What action must you take? For example, should you call the doctor or take certain extra medicine? You are now managing your own health along with your doctor's help. Chapters 5 and 6 can help you to plan more specifically on how to manage to "stay healthy" and work to prevent another stroke.

Are There Restrictions in the Use of Alcohol?

Alcohol is a drug that works on the brain. In some persons, it can actually cause strokes. The effects of alcohol even on normal people can cause a lack of balance and slurred speech. For persons that have had brain injury from stroke, it is likely that alcohol can affect their performance even more than in a person who has not suffered a stroke. One patient who experienced problems with balance after his stroke found that he would fall. He could no longer have his usual drink with his dinner for fear of falling. Even one beer was more than he could manage. One way to think about this warning is that you need every possible nerve call to be working at top efficiency for you to carry on your life. Using drugs like alcohol can push you over the edge and make it harder for you to do what you can ordinarily do only with difficulty.

Exercise 2.4 Asking Questions/Getting Answers

This exercise can help to review the questions you could have asked. Check off those that you have had answered to your satisfaction and then define other questions you may want to ask.

_____ 1. When will I be independent?

_____ 2. What recovery can I expect?

_____ 3. How we deal with changes in our relationship?

_____ 4. What about sex?

_____ 5. How to deal with feelings about myself, self image?

_____ 6. How can I get around?

_____ 7. Can I get back to work?

_____ 8. How can I prevent another stroke?

_____ 9. Are there restrictions on use of alcohol?

Are there other questions that you now want to ask? List them below and try to get the answers.

_____

_____

_____

_____

—3—

Understanding Your Health Plan

GERBEN DEJONG
PHILLIP W. BEATTY

Now more than ever before in U.S. history, health insurance influences the types and amount of health care services we receive. Unlike in decades past, our health-insurance plans profoundly affect our choices of doctors, hospitals, and other providers, as well as our access to care. Managed care—the predominant form of health insurance today—has transformed the health-insurance industry, including Medicare, and introduced us to concepts such as gatekeepers, preferred-provider organizations, and point-of-service options.

As a health care consumer who may be faced with the aftermath of stroke, it is important to educate yourself about your own or your loved one's health-insurance plan and the services it covers. By becoming an informed consumer, you will be more prepared to navigate the insurance system and more empowered to get the most for your health-plan dollar. Furthermore, expressing your views about your health-insurance plan may influence constructive changes in the plan that will benefit others who are affected by stroke or other serious medical problems.

This chapter provides an overview of the types of health-insurance coverage that are available and the types of insurers that offer coverage. It also includes a list of important questions to ask about your health-insurance plan as it relates to health care following stroke and provides advice for people faced with denials of coverage. We begin this chapter by describing the major types of health plans that are available. We then describe the major health-plan providers, including the Medicare and Medicaid programs.

TYPES OF HEALTH-INSURANCE PLANS

Health-insurance plans can be placed in one of two broad categories: fee-for-service plans and managed-care plans. Generally, fee-for-service plans offer greater flexibility in choosing physicians, hospitals, and other providers, while managed-care plans offer the benefits of lower out-of-pocket costs and less paperwork.

Fee-for-Service Plans

Traditional health-insurance plans, known as "fee-for-service" or "indemnity" plans, pay the physician, hospital, or other provider a fee for each covered service that is rendered. In such plans, you can go to any physician, hospital, or other health-care provider that accepts the plan's payment, and the insurance company will pay a percentage of the charges for all covered benefits. As recently as the mid-1970s, most people with health insurance in this country were covered by fee-for-service policies. Today, however, fewer than half of insured persons have fee-for-service coverage.

In addition to paying premiums, fee-for-service policyholders usually are responsible for some of the costs of covered services that are rendered. First, you may have to pay an annual deductible for each individual or for the entire family before the insurance company pays any benefits on your behalf. You must pay this deductible (such as $250 or $500) each year before the policy pays for any benefits. Generally, the higher the deductible the lower your annual, quarterly, or monthly premiums, and the lower the deductible the higher the premiums.

Second, after you have met the deductible, you may have to pay co-insurance, which is a percentage of the "usual and customary" charge (or "reasonable and customary" charge) for the covered service. This charge is the prevailing cost of the service in your geographic area. Often, the insurance policy pays 80 percent of the usual and customary charge and the policyholder pays co-insurance of 20 percent of the charge. If your provider charges more than the usual and customary amount, then you must pay the difference in addition to the co-insurance. Most fee-for-service plans pay the full amount of hospital expenses, although some require 20 percent co-insurance.

Most fee-for-service policies set a maximum for out-of-pocket expenses (expenses that you, the policyholder, pay). After you have reached this maximum amount in a calendar year, the plan pays 100 percent of the usual and customary charges for covered benefits, and you no longer pay the co-insurance. Fee-for-service plans also may set a lifetime coverage limit—typically at least $1 million.

Insurance companies offer two kinds of fee-for-service coverage, basic and major medical, that sometimes are combined into a single "comprehensive plan." Basic coverage is used toward the costs of a hospital room and care received in the hospital, including some hospital services and supplies (for example, X-rays and prescribed medicine), as well as the costs of physician visits and inpatient and outpatient surgery. Major medical coverage provides protection above that offered by basic coverage and covers costs associated with long-term, high-cost illnesses and injuries.

Fee-for-service policies offer the greatest freedom in selecting health-care providers and do not require physician referrals or authorizations (although certain procedures may need to be pre-certified, or pre-approved). However, out-of-pocket expenses often are higher for fee-for-service policies than for managed-care plans, and, unlike with managed-care plans, you may need to fill out and submit claim forms to the insurance company.

Managed-Care Plans

More than half of all Americans who have health insurance today are enrolled in managed-care plans, which now number more than 600 nationwide. Managed-care plans deliver comprehensive health care services at a reduced price for members, who, in most plans, agree to use providers in the plan's network. The physicians, hospitals, and other providers in the plan's network have negotiated fees and contracts with the plan. Managed-care plans once were offered only through private health-insurance companies. Today, they also are offered through the government's Medicare and Medicaid programs, as described below.

In recent years, managed care has changed patterns of stroke care by decreasing the number of days patients stay in the acute-care hospital setting and by shifting rehabilitation placement away from inpatient hospital settings and toward sub-acute settings such as nursing homes. These apparent effects of managed care vary according to factors such as the level of managed care's presence in a particular geographic area.

In managed-care plans, you pay a flat premium amount in advance. This premium pays for all covered services, whether or not you use the plan's services and regardless of how many services you use. However, you probably have to pay a small co-payment for some services (such as $10 for a physician office visit or $5 for a medication prescription) and, in some cases, you may have to pay co-insurance. Out-of-pocket expenses typically are lower in managed-care plans than in fee-for-service plans, but the choice of health care providers, facilities, and services usually is more limited.

Health maintenance organizations (HMOs) are the oldest form of managed-care plan. Since HMOs were introduced, other types of plans combining features of both traditional fee-for-service policies and managed-care plans have emerged. These hybrid plans include "preferred- provider organizations" and "point-of-service" options, which offer financial incentives for using providers in the plan's network, but are less restrictive than traditional HMOs.

It is important to recognize that the distinctions among health-insurance plan types are becoming increasingly blurred, not only among managed-care plans but also between managed- care and fee-for-service plans. Many managed-care plans now include traditional fee-for-service plan features, while many fee-for-service plans now use managed-care methods of containing costs and ensuring the appropriateness of care. This evolution has resulted in greater choice for consumers.

Health Maintenance Organizations

HMOs are one specific type of managed care. These plans offer members comprehensive health- care services, including preventive care, in return for monthly premiums and usually small co-payments (such as $5, $10, or $15) that are paid directly to the provider at the time of service. Typically, HMOs require neither deductibles nor co-insurance, and sometimes they do not require co-payments. HMO members receive their medical care at either a central medical facility (in staff model HMOs) or, more commonly, at the private offices of participating doctors (in group model HMOs or individual practice associations).

As an HMO member, you select a primary-care physician from within the plan's network. For adults, this physician typically is an internist or a family-practice doctor. Your primary-care physician coordinates the care you receive and serves as a "gatekeeper" by providing referrals to other providers. In HMO plans, you must receive a referral from your primary-care provider to see a medical specialist, such as a neurologist.

HMOs offer members the advantages of not having to submit claims to the insurance company for services received and having lower out-of-pocket expenses than in fee-for-service policies—an advantage if you see physicians or use other providers frequently. However, your choice of health care providers is more limited, and your access to providers is more restricted.

Point-of-Service Options

A growing number of HMOs now offer point-of-service (POS) options, which provide financial incentives to members choosing network providers while allowing members to use non-network providers. With POS options, a primary-care physician coordinates your care, usually making referrals to other providers in the network. If your primary-care physician makes a referral outside of the network, then the insurer pays most or all of the costs. However, you must pay co-insurance if you refer yourself to a non-network provider. Thus, a POS option increases the flexibility of your managed-care plan by giving you more choices of providers.

Flexibility in selecting providers may be particularly important if you need access to individual specialists, such as neurologists or rehabilitation physicians, who do not participate in the HMO plan. The trade-offs are that POS premiums are higher than HMO premiums, and that you must pay a larger deductible than in an HMO.

Preferred Provider Organizations

More than 89 million Americans are enrolled in preferred provider organizations (PPOs), which far outnumber HMOs. Like POS options, PPOs combine the features of HMOs with those of traditional fee-for-service health-insurance plans. PPOs offer members financial incentives for choosing health-care providers from within the plan's network. If you visit a network physician, you pay a co-payment at the time of service. For some services, you may have to pay a deductible and co-insurance. If you visit a non-network provider, you must meet a deductible and pay co-insurance. You may also be responsible for any difference between the amount the provider charges and the amount the plan will pay.

PPOs most often do not use primary-care physicians to coordinate plan members' care. PPO physicians may make referrals, but plan members can refer themselves to physicians, including physicians outside the plan. Therefore, members are free to use any physician without prior approval.

Long-Term Care Insurance

Long-term care insurance plans are available to cover the costs of services that may be needed over an extended period of time. The costs of these policies vary as do the services they cover and their limits of coverage. Most long-term care insurance policies pay a set dollar amount for each day you receive covered care in a nursing home or at home. It is difficult to obtain long-term care insurance after your need for long-term care services has begun.

Unless you are fortunate enough to have a long-term care insurance policy in place, you may not be covered for long-term expenses associated with nursing-home care, long-term in-home services and supports, or other assistance that you may need after a stroke. Private health insurance and Medicare coverage of long-term care is limited. For example, Medicare coverage is limited to 100 days of skilled nursing care per episode of care. If after 100 days you still need long-term services and supports (often non-medical), you must pay out-of-pocket for those services. You may also qualify for long-term care services if you are eligible for Medicaid, described in the next section of this chapter.

Talk with your medical social worker about your options for financing long-term care if it is needed.

TYPES OF PAYERS

Fee-for-service and managed-care health-insurance plans are offered through private insurers, as well as through the Medicare and Medicaid programs.

Figure 3.1 Questions to Ask About Your Health-insurance Plan

After a stroke, you will want to make the most of your health-insurance dollars. To do so, you must develop a clear understanding of what the plan covers and how it works. Remember, while many plans are similar, the details of each plan are unique.

Begin by reading the plan's member handbook and the policy itself to educate yourself about the benefits, coverage, and limits on coverage. Take notes and write down any questions you have. If you need assistance understanding the plan, call the insurance company for clarification, talk with your physician's office staff or your hospital's financial services office, or consult your employer's health benefits officer (if applicable).

At a minimum, you should know the answers to the following questions:

Overall Coverage

- Does the plan set a limit, or "cap" on the maximum dollar amount that will be paid each year or over the insured person's lifetime?
- Does the plan have "catastrophic limits of coverage," which determine the maximum out-of-pocket expenses you must pay for medical services and prescription drugs?
- What is the amount of the annual deductible, if any?
- What co-payments or co-insurance amounts are required for services that will be needed?
- Does the plan limit coverage of pre-existing conditions?

Physician Services

- Does the plan require a primary-care physician's referral for specialist care?
- What co-payment or co-insurance amount must be paid for each visit to a physician?

Hospital Care

- Does the plan pay the full amount of hospital care, including room and board, and services and supplies (such as surgery, X-rays, and prescribed medications)?
- Does the plan place a limit on the number of hospital days covered?

Rehabilitation Services

- Does the plan pay for rehabilitation services, such as physical therapy, occupational therapy, and speech-language pathology?
- What limits are set on the number of rehabilitation visits or the number of days that rehabilitation services will be provided?

Skilled Nursing Care

- Does the plan pay for skilled nursing care in a nursing home if needed?
- If skilled nursing care is covered, must it be prescribed following a hospital stay?

Custodial Care

- Does the plan pay for custodial care? Custodial care primarily helps with daily needs (for example, eating, bathing, and dressing) but does not require treat-

Figure 3.1 Questions to Ask About Your Health-insurance Plan (Continued)

---

ment or services from specially trained professionals such as doctors, nurses, and therapists.
- What limits are set on custodial care?

Home Health Care
- Does the plan cover home health care services?
- Is there a limit on the number of home health care days or visits that are covered (for example, 90 days or 90 visits)?

Medical Equipment
- Does the plan pay for medically necessary equipment, such as walkers, wheelchairs, and special beds?
- If the plan pays for medical equipment, what portion of the cost is covered?
- Does the plan pay for the initial purchase as well as replacement equipment, or only for the initial purchase?

Prescription Drugs
- Does the plan pay for prescription drugs?
- Is there an annual dollar "cap" on coverage of prescription drugs?
- If prescription drugs are covered, do you need to pay a co-payment? How much is the co-payment (for example, $10 per prescription)?

Emergency Care
- Does the plan pay for hospital emergency room care
- If so, how is such care defined
- Under what circumstances is emergency room care *not* covered (for example, visits that are "false alarms

---

Medicare

Medicare, the nation's largest health-insurance program, serves more than 39 million Americans and is the most important source of health care coverage for people with stroke. Administered by the Health Care Financing Administration (HCFA), an agency within the U.S. Department of Health and Human Services, Medicare provides health insurance to people age 65 and over, some people with disabilities, and people who have end-stage renal disease (permanent kidney failure). If you are eligible for Social Security or Railroad Retirement benefits and are age 65, then you and your spouse automatically qualify for Medicare.

Medicare has two parts: Part A (hospital insurance) and Part B (medical insurance). Part A helps pay for the costs of hospital and skilled nursing facility stays, home health care, and hospice care. Part B helps pay for physician services; outpatient hospital care; physical, occupational, and speech therapy; diagnostic tests; durable medical equipment; home health care; and other services. If you are eligible for Medicare, no premium is required for Part A, but you must pay a premium for Part B. Although Medicare pays for many health expenses, the program does not cover all services, including most nursing-home care, long-term care services in the home, and prescription drugs.

The Balanced Budget Act of 1997 (Public Law 105-33) enacted the most important changes in the Medicare and Medicaid programs since the programs were established in 1965. One of the most notable changes was the creation of Medicare+Choice, which gives Medicare participants the opportunity to choose the "Original Medicare Plan" or to enroll in a Medicare managed-care plan. This law, in essence, shifted the federal government's role as a payer of health services to that of a sponsor of health plans.

The number of Medicare managed-care enrollees grew rapidly between 1994 and 1998. The proportion of Medicare managed-care plan members jumped from 9 percent to 15 percent. However, Medicare beneficiary enrollment in managed-care plans varies greatly from region to region, and Medicare managed-care plans are not available in all areas of the country.

To be eligible for the new Medicare managed-care option, you must participate in both Part A and Part B, and you must not have end-stage renal disease. Medicare managed-care plans include HMOs; HMOs with POS options; PPOs; and provider-sponsored organizations (PSOs) (HMOs offered by groups of hospitals and doctors). Medicare managed-care plans offer attractive features, particularly for young, healthy beneficiaries, but they also have the same disadvantages as non-Medicare managed-care plans. For example, your choice of specialists may be restricted, and use of some services, particularly expensive services, may be carefully scrutinized.

The Original Medicare Plan is the traditional, fee-for-service Medicare system and is available to all Medicare beneficiaries nationwide. As in any other fee-for-service plan, in the Original Medicare Plan, you may go to any doctor, hospital, or other health care provider, although the provider must agree to accept Medicare payment. You pay a deductible and co-insurance, as well as costs that exceed Medicare's allowable charges, up to a pre-set limit.

Those who choose the Original Medicare Plan have the option of purchasing Part B (medical insurance) for an additional premium. In addition, they may purchase a private supplemental insurance policy, called a Medigap policy, that covers some of the expenses that the Original Medicare Plan does not. Medigap policies must cover certain expenses, such as the daily co-insurance amount for hospitalization, and some plans may cover such services as preventive medical care and prescription drugs. Ten standard Medigap policy types, designated by the letters A through J, are available. However, all 10 types are not sold in all states; only Plan A must be made available to all Medicare recipients. One type of Medigap policy, called Medicare SELECT, may require you to use doctors or hospitals within the plan's network in order for you to be eligible for full benefits; this type of policy generally has a lower premium than a regular Medigap policy.

Medicare also has a trial program through which some beneficiaries have the option of having a medical savings account (MSA). With MSAs, beneficiaries can shelter income in a tax-free account to pay for medical expenses. Unlike other Medicare health plans, there are no limits on what providers can charge people with MSAs above the amount paid by the MSA plan. In addition, the deductible for an MSA plan can be considerably higher than with other Medicare plans.

Medicaid

The Medicaid program provides health-insurance coverage for low-income individuals and families, as well as for people with certain kinds of disabilities. This program is a jointly funded cooperative venture between the federal government and state governments. It is designed to assist states in providing adequate medical care to eligible persons. Each state administers its own program, and rules for Medicare eligibility and coverage differ from state to state. To receive federal matching funds, each state must cover a set of basic services such as inpatient and outpatient hospital care, physician services, laboratory and X-ray services, and nursing facility services for persons ages 21 or older. States may also cover many other services, including rehabilitation services, prescription drugs, and personal care services.

Health care providers that participate in Medicaid receive payments directly and agree to accept the Medicaid reimbursement as payment in full. However, states may ask Medicaid recipients to pay nominal deductibles, co-insurance, or co-payments.

Medicaid is the largest insurer of long-term care for all Americans. This program covers 68 percent of nursing-home residents and more than 50 percent of nursing-home costs. Although most long-term care spending is for institutional care, Medicaid is working toward shifting the delivery of services to home and community settings. Many people choose to reduce, or "spend down," their assets in order to qualify for Medicaid and receive coverage for nursing-home care. This approach, however, requires careful advance planning over a period of years.

If you are elderly and meet the income requirements, your state's Medicaid program may help pay for your Medicare premiums and some of your out-of-pocket Medicare expenses. In addition, if you are eligible for full Medicaid coverage, your state's Medicaid program will supplement your Medicare coverage by paying for services and supplies, such as nursing-home care beyond the 100-day Medicare limit and prescription drugs, that are available under Medicaid.

One of the most significant trends in the Medicaid program in recent years has been the rapid growth in managed-care enrollment among Medicaid recipients. This trend results in part from the states' authority under current law to launch a variety of new programs, including expanding managed-care enrollment. Between 1993 and 1998, the percentage of Medicare recipients enrolled in managed-care plans nationally climbed from 14 percent to 54 percent.

Private Insurance

Health insurance is available through a variety of private entities, including not-for-profit organizations and for-profit companies. These organizations offer a wide range of fee-for-service and managed-care plans, including group plans (such as those provided through employers and unions) and individual plans. Each insurer's plans differ from other those of other insurers, and policies offered by the same insurer may differ from one another.

Figure 3.2 What to Do When Coverage Is Denied?

Coping with the physical, emotional, and psychological effects of stroke is challenging and often frustrating for both the stroke survivor and loved ones. But many stroke survivors also are faced with financial challenges, including those associated with health insurance. Although you may be focused on stroke recovery and rehabilitation, it is important to be sure that you are getting the most for your health-insurance dollar—and to know your health-insurance rights, particularly when faced with denials of payment by a private insurer or Medicare

What should you do if you believe that your insurer has unfairly denied coverage for a particular service? Below are some tips for resolving or appealing denials of coverage.

Know your policy. Begin by understanding what your private insurance policy or Medicare does and does not cover. When you enrolled in the plan, you should have received an explanation of your benefits, the plan's exclusion policies, and the plan's appeal procedures, including the appeals-process timetable. If a service is not covered by your plan, then an appeal will likely be fruitless. You may obtain information about Medicare coverage from the Health Care Financing Administration (HCFA) (see resource list).

Consult with your employer. If your insurance is purchased through an employer, talk with the health-insurance benefits officer to ensure that you understand the plan's coverage and to ask for advice on how to handle your situation. Your benefits officer may contact the insurer on your behalf or may help you to contact the insurer's service representative to clarify your coverage.

Call member services. If you have a private insurance policy, ask the insurer's member services department for information about your policy's coverage of the service in question. This department may be able to resolve the problem without your having to file a formal appeal.

Understand the appeals process. Learn as much as possible about your insurer's grievance or appeals process. This process, which differs from plan to plan, is designed to review denials of coverage to determine whether specific denials are valid. The insurance plan materials and the member services department should provide information about this process.

Act quickly. If you choose to appeal a denial of coverage, be sure to file the appeal within the time period allowed by the plan (for example, one to two months from the date you are notified of a denial of coverage). Request an expedited review if you need the medical service urgently.

Put it in writing. If you decide to file a grievance or appeal, do it in writing and send it by registered mail.

Keep a paper trail. Make a copy of all correspondence you send, and file it with correspondence from the insurance company. Also, keep a log documenting your conversations regarding your claim. Be sure to make a note of the names, job titles, departments, and telephone numbers of people with whom you spoke.

Enlist the support of your physician. Ask your doctor to write a letter to the insurance company that clearly explains why the treatment was necessary. Additional

Figure 3.2 What to Do When Coverage Is Denied? (Continued)

information about the "medical necessity" of the service may help the insurer to resolve the problem.

Talk with state officials. Find out about any state laws and regulations that apply to your situation. You may wish to file a complaint with your state's insurance bureau if you continue to believe that the denial of coverage is unfair. You may also want to ask your legislators for advice and support.

Good News for Consumers

Nearly all health maintenance organizations (HMOs) allow members to appeal decisions denying payment for services, but often the reviews are handled internally by employees of the insurance company—who may be partial to the company's interests. But today there is good news for consumers.

At least 18 states now have laws giving consumers the right to have appeals reviewed by external panels of experts, at least for plans that are regulated by the individual states. In addition, beginning in the year 2000, HMOs seeking a stamp of approval by the National Committee on Quality Assurance, the HMO accrediting body, must provide plan members the right to appeal denials to a panel of external experts. Even the HMO trade group, the American Association of Health Plans, supports the idea of external appeals panels to help protect plan members from unfair denials of payment for care.

In addition to setting limits on individual covered benefits, many private fee-for-service and managed-care plans set limits, called "caps," on the dollar amount that will be paid each year or over a person's lifetime. On the other hand, most private health-insurance policies and plans have catastrophic limits of coverage. These limits place a ceiling on the out-of-pocket expenses that you must pay for medical services and prescription drugs. The limits include any premiums, deductibles, and co-payments that you have contributed toward your care. Fee-for-service plans generally set higher catastrophic limits of coverage than those set by managed-care plans.

Most private health-insurance plans cover skilled nursing care received in a nursing home, as long as it is prescribed following a hospital stay. However, custodial care received in a nursing home, long-term care facility, or at home generally is not covered by private health-insurance plans. Custodial care is care provided mainly to help patients take care of their daily needs (eating, bathing, and dressing) and does not require treatment or services from specially trained professionals, such as doctors, therapists, or nurses.

Figure 3.3 Important Cost-Containment Features of Health-Insurance Plans

Fee-for service and managed-care health-insurance plans differ in many ways, but to-day they also share certain features that are designed to contain health care costs. Sometimes these features do not seem to be in the patient's best interest, but they do exist and it is important to be aware of them as you negotiate the health care system following stroke. These features include utilization review, preauthorization of services, and discharge planning.

Utilization review is a process through which a health-insurance company determines whether specific medical or surgical services ordered by a physician are appropriate or "medically necessary" (although health-insurance plans differ in their definitions of medical necessity). Utilization review can take place either before or after the patient receives the service.

Preauthorization of services is a requirement for pre-approval from the health-insurance company for most non-emergency hospital admissions, surgical procedures, and other expensive procedures.

Discharge planning takes place when the patient is in an acute-care or rehabilitation hospital setting. This type of planning helps to ensure that the patient is transferred to an appropriate, cost-effective setting, such as skilled nursing facility, for continued care if needed.

A FINAL WORD

Whether you participate in Medicare, have a private health-insurance plan, or receive Medicaid benefits, understanding health-insurance today can be challenging, particularly when coupled with the other challenges you may be experiencing following a stroke. By educating yourself about your plan and the services it covers, you will be better prepared to make decisions about your health care and to make the most of your insurance dollars. If you have questions about your plan, talk with your medical social worker, the patient financial services office at your hospital, your doctor, or your insurer's member-services department.

Special thanks to Susan R. Farrer, M.A., for her contributions to the preparation of this chapter. Ms. Farrer is a writing and editorial consultant who specializes in health and medical topics.

4

Planning to Strike Back at Stroke

BRENDAN E. CONROY
MARK N. OZER

TAKING CHARGE OF YOUR LIFE

For most people, having a stroke is one of the worst things that ever happened to them. Suddenly one can no longer control one's body, and especially troubling for most people is the loss of control of an arm and/or leg. The simple acts of reaching for a glass of water or getting out of bed are hard, if not impossible. One must re-learn what had been done without even thinking. At times, it seems nearly impossible to carry on. This loss of control of the body is due to damage to the brain. The brain not only controls your body parts but also organizes the ways of responding to people and deciding how to deal with change throughout life. On top of the loss of control of one's body comes a loss of control of one's life. For most people, the stroke brought them into a hospital, and that brings its own frustrations. Even in the best hospitals, response to a call bell may sometimes be slow. The need for others to care for you and the inability to deal with your own needs can lead to constant frustration and sometimes anger.

You can call both upon yourself and upon others to help you to deal with the stroke. At first, you may need others to care for you, to help with your physical needs and to lift and move you. Even then, the energy to move cannot come entirely from others. You can still use whatever strength you have to contribute. This individual contribution must also come from you and from your own directions. As you ask someone else to help, you should also be commanding yourself to do a part of the work.

The energy must come from within yourself as well as from others.

75

Others, such as your therapists and nurses, can help you by giving you instructions about how to overcome some of your stroke-related problems—for example, how to get out of bed, how to dress yourself once again, and how to prevent another stroke. The way to accomplish these activities may be different from before. You will need to learn these new instructions and repeat them to yourself. While giving the instructions to yourself, you can change them and make them more your own. In the long run, you are the best one to figure out what works for you. They also work better because you, better than someone else, can give yourself just the right instructions at just the right time

MAKING PLANS FOR YOURSELF

There are planning questions that you can think about and answer to the best of your ability. This planning process will help you work through the stroke recovery process. These planning questions can help you to take charge of your life again. By making a plan, reviewing it, and revising it as needed, you can regain a greater degree of independence and control of your life. You may have worked on self-improvement without really needing to think about it before the stroke. Now, just like relearning how to get out of bed, self-improvement may need to be relearned and may perhaps become even better than before your stroke. You will also get better results as you become more aware that they are your results, that you did it. You will recognize that you can still make a difference in your life by realizing that you have set goals, accomplished them, seen what works, and continue to reach even higher goals.

You may see this self-help happening in many different areas. The most obvious area for you to see this positive change is in regaining control of your bodily functions, such as blood pressure, and your urine and bowel movements. At the same time, you can begin to regain control of moving around, dressing, taking care of yourself and many other aspects of your life. The questions we will ask can help in all aspects of your life . . . help you in "adding life to years."

The Questions We Will Be Asking

- What are my problems?
- What do I want to see happen?

- What results have I had?
- How did I get those results?

These questions can help you tap into our own thoughts and strengths. Tapping into your own thoughts is a way of being introspective—looking into yourself. Looking into yourself may be hard for some people. Putting these thoughts into words can be quite challenging. Words may not come easily after a stroke. But, even persons with problems in communication due to their stroke can show their agreement to ideas suggested by others. They can shake their heads or say "yes" or "no."

The professionals on your rehabilitation team will try to help you understand your problems, what you might be able to do about these problems, and finally what might be goals that are worth working on. The doctor, nurses, and therapists on your team will ask for your agreement. It is your responsibility as well as your right to let the team know if you agree or disagree with their goals for you. The staff in turn have their own rights and responsibilities. They have a high degree of training and expertise. They have experience predicting what you might need. You are an individual, and only you may know in the long run what you really need. You have had experience with yourself in dealing with problems in the past. The best result would be to use your experience and that of your team members to decide together how to plan for your rehabilitation .

This chapter illustrates how to use the planning questions. The four basic questions that were listed above should be answered by each person in terms of his/her own individual needs. Each of the chapters in the rest of this book explores an area of potential problems. Within each chapter there may be subjects of great importance to you. For example, almost everyone who has experienced a stroke would be concerned about preventing another stroke. Some, however, have a particular interest in managing their high blood pressure while others are concerned about the use of blood thinners. These medications prevent clots that could go to the brain and cause another stroke.

Each of the divisions within each of the next two chapters (5 and 6) dealing with your health and stroke prevention follows the same pattern. The problems are identified, followed by a discussion of what worked to help other patients with the same problem. The third part of each division contains a log sheet to use to help you make your own plan to deal with your own specific problem. Now that you have learned to make a plan for yourself in the chapters on "Staying Healthy" and "Prevention of Stroke," you can use that same format for making a plan for yourself in the chapters on "Medical Rehabilitation." In these other chapters, the log sheet is at the end of each chapter. Table 4.1 illustrates the log sheet at the end of each chapter.

What are your problems?

You can use a check-off system to identify the problems covered in Chapters 5 and 6. In the other chapters, you can identify the problems for yourself. These problems include: What are your goals? What progress have you made up to now? What worked to achieve that progress? Sometimes what you did to achieve goals in one area can be applied to new goals. The little boxes on the log sheet can record which answers to questions came from you and which from the therapist or nurse.

WHO IS DOING THE TALKING?

Who is answering the questions? It is your responsibility to contribute to the solutions of your problems. Your contributions have the closest connection with you, what you think, and what you need.

Table 4.2 describes how much the answers are yours. Are you coming up with answers to any of the questions being asked? This is called a "Statement"response. You are making a statement about what you think. You can put an "S" in the little box on your log. This mark means that you have good awareness of yourself, of your problems, of your goals, of your successes, and of what you do that works. It may be easier for you to answer certain questions than others. You may be better able to make a "Statement" about your "status" which we term how well you are doing at this time. It may be harder for you to make a "Statement" about your future in answering the question of GOALS which simply asks what you want to see happen. The rehabilitation team members will try to give you some ideas for goals and what they think might work to which you can give "Agreement." When you have

Table 4.1 Making a Plan for Myself

1. What are my problems?

The answers to the question and the problems are yours to describe. The problem you may have depends on your own particular situation and your concerns.

1. _____
2. _____
3. _____

The answers to the question of goals are also yours to describe. It is helpful not only to specify what you wish to accomplish, but how much, or how fast, or how independently. When answering the question about what results you find have been achieved, it is helpful to specify not only what the results were but where or when it happened. The answers to the question about what works may also be your ideas or equipment you have found useful. It is helpful not only to specify what you do to contribute to the results, but how you go about it. "How often" or "where" or "when" are some additional questions to help make your statements more specific.

2. Following my plan

Participation: Agreement (A) Confirmed Agreement (CA) Statement (S) Specific Statement (SS)			
Date	**Status/Progress**	**Goals**	**What Works**
	☐	☐	☐
	☐	☐	☐
	☐	☐	☐
	☐	☐	☐

Table 4.2 Who is Doing the Talking

	Therapist	Patient
Statement	Asks questions	Answers for himself
Confirmed Agreement	Offers ideas	Agrees and puts into own words
Agreement	Offers ideas	Agrees (or disagrees) "Yes" or "No"

a chance to say "yes" or "no" to an idea made by others, you are agreeing that they have a good idea for you. This is the "Agreement " level. You can put an "A" in the little box on the log sheet. You can think about this as being "true" or "false." When you were in school, it was easier to say "true" or "false" than to come up with answers on your own. At this agreement level many discussions occur between patients and health professionals. For example, your nurse or therapist may recommend some goals to you or some ideas how to accomplish those goals.

An intermediate level is to put the therapist's suggestion into your own words. This is considered a "Confirmed Agreement" response. You can put "CA" in the little box on your log sheet. You have a chance to say what you think about an idea originally coming from another person. If you were to say it aloud, it becomes even more your idea. You can, as many people do, change your thoughts when you put them into your own words. You can also hear it for yourself. This step is an important one. For example, in answer to the question about what worked to control your hypertension, you can mention your medication. Once you tell someone else what it is, you can be clearer about it yourself.

Once you have reached the level of making a "Statement," answering for yourself, you can then try to make it clearer. Becoming clearer can be measured by the amount of detail you put into your statements. For example, you can describe not only what medications you take, but also how much you take in terms of dosage, and when you take them. You can also describe your answers to the other questions in terms of not only "what," but "when," and "how much." You can put "SS" in the little box in your log sheet. This is considered a "Specific Statement" response. It means that you are clear about your answers. For example, the clearer you are about what you are trying to accomplish, the more likely you are to get there and the more likely you are to know when you have gotten there.

HOW TO USE THE LOG SHEET

For example, during your first OT planning session in Table 4-3, you and your OT will agree on what activities, such as feeding yourself or dressing yourself, that you may now able to do. For example, you may be able to do 50 percent of your own bathing and 75 percent of putting on your shirt. This would be written in the STATUS box . Under GOALS, you might decide to work on doing 75 percent of your bathing and 90 percent of putting on your shirt over the course of the next week Table 4.3 illustrates that first planning session. The little box reflects who does the talking. You are in "agreement" with the ideas presented by the OT with an "A" in each of the little boxes.

A week later, at the second planning session, you would indicate under STATUS if the goals had been met and what was accomplished, even if it is not the same as you had planned on. You agree with the therapist that "75 percent of the bathing" was accomplished. You go even further in being able to put what was said into your own words (CA). You could then consider the question WHAT WORKED: how did you accomplish what happened? You agree (A) with the therapist that what may have worked is using a long-handled sponge to wash the hard to-reach parts of your body. You also agree ("A") with the therapist that it was helpful "to know my goal." You agree (A) with the therapist that you have improved in putting on a shirt but not to 90 percent yet. You say ("S") that what prevented you from getting beyond 80 percent of putting on your shirt was pain in your involved shoulder. You put this information under WHAT WORKED/Problems.

In setting your GOAL for the next planning session, you agree ("A") once again to go for 90 percent of putting on your shirt. But your plan would include doing something about the pain in your shoulder by massage and stretching exercises. During this planning session, you have begun to do some of the talking by going beyond "Agreement" for a few parts of the discussion.

At the third session, you can assess your STATUS once again in terms of putting on your shirt. You did meet your goal and you say that on your own ("S"). For WHAT WORKED, you agree and put into your own words ("CA") that you reduced the pain by exercise. Now you have a clear idea that the massage and stretching you did with the therapist can help reduce the pain, even if it remains some-

Table 4.3 Planning Sessions

Participation: Agreement (A) Confirmed Agreement (CA) Statement (S) Specific Statement (SS)			
Date	**Status/Progress**	**Goals**	**What Worked/Problems**
08/01	A — I can do: 50 percent of my own bathing	A — 75 percent of my own bathing	☐
	A — 75 percent of putting a shirt on	A — 90 percent of putting a shirt on	☐
08/08	CA — I can do: 7 percent of my own bathing	A — 90 percent of my own bathing	A — Use a long handled sponge A — Knowing my goal
	A — 80 percent of putting a shirt on (not met yet)	A — Reduce shoulder pain and do 90 percent of putting a shirt on	S — Shoulder pain
08/15	S — 90 percent of putting a shirt on	☐	CA — Reduced shoulder pain with stretching and massage.
	CA — I need 50 percent help to get in/out of bath tub.	CA — Only need 25 percent help for bath tub transfers	S — Knowing my goal

what troublesome. You can now consider a new area: getting in and out of the bathtub. You would record the present STATUS and GOAL by putting into your own words ("CA") the ideas offered by the therapists. Now that you have had experience in accomplishing the other goals, you could use some of the ideas about what worked in dealing with this next problem. One thing that you know worked for you was "knowing my goal." You realize that knowing the goal of "25 percent help for tub transfers" can help you get to that level of progress. If you know what you are trying to achieve, it's easier to get it done.

This review process can be used again and again to determine the degree of progress, those things that worked or interfered with progress, and the setting of new goals for yourself. During in-patient rehabilitation, it is customary for your team to have a weekly Team Conference to discuss your status, goals, and successes. Your log sheet gives you the chance to keep up with the planning being done. It is particularly helpful if you are there to participate in the team conference. The log sheet gives you a way to keep even better track of what is discussed at the conference.

Review of your status and goal in managing your blood pressure or blood sugar is another important area of concern. Many people who have had a stroke have high blood pressure. This problem is one of the most important areas you can work on to protect yourself from having another stroke. Your doctor or nurse will tell you what the goal is. You can and should ask why the blood pressure goal is set where it is. This can vary with your age and other factors. It is a relatively easy set of numbers to remember, but it is very important that you know the desired blood pressure level. You can write it down or have the nurse write it down so that you can remember it. A nurse will generally check your blood pressure. Each time the nurse measures your blood pressure, ask for the result and evaluate if the levels are meeting the goal set by your doctor or nurse.

After you go home, you will be doing the same thing. You can learn how to check your own blood pressure. It is easier than you might think with some of the automatic machines available. It is important to know if you are meeting your goal. If you are meeting your blood pressure goal, you can think about your actions that help. If you are not meeting your goal, that means that your blood pressure is uncontrolled. You need to discuss it with your primary-care physician. Eventually, you might be able to figure out for yourself what you could do in addition to taking your medicine. You can read more information about controlling your blood pressure in Chapter 5.

Reliving successes, as important as they are, is not enough. You need to know how the successes happened so that you can experience more of them. Even more important, you need to ask yourself "What did I do to make those successes happen?" The purpose of this question is to discover what worked. Then you can make improvements and assess your actions that may have helped. These actions may be repeatable to make more progress.

Many people believe that they have nothing to do with getting a medical condition such as high blood pressure under control. When a person with high blood pressure achieves better control and is staying under their goal, the person may credit medication for the result. However, the result comes from the person taking the pills and letting them work inside one's body. You agreed to take the pills as directed, and you became healthier. The doctor or nurse did not stand over you to force you to take the pills. You took them as you had agreed with the doctor. It was your action that worked.

The next chapters of this book are discussions of problems that many stroke survivors have and suggestions on how to work through them. It is hoped that you will have many successes on your path to recovery. Planning for yourself along with the professionals on your team can help you to regain a sense of control over your body and your life. It is the best way to "strike back at stroke."

5

Staying Healthy

FATEMEH MILANI
MARK N. OZER

WHAT ARE THE PROBLEMS?

Problems with your health can affect the ability to recover from the effects of a stroke. They can interfere with the rehabilitation process. In fact, the stroke itself may be responsible for the problems you may have in health. The stroke affects not only your mobility, sensation, and vision as well as your thinking, but it also affects other systems of your body. A major problem for a person who has had a stroke is regaining control of bodily functions enabling a healthy life. The chapter discusses issues of maintaining adequate nutrition and satisfactory bowel and bladder function possibly compromised in persons with stroke. Also covered are central post-stroke pain syndrome, musculoskeletal pain (joints and muscles pain) and shoulder hand syndrome (painful shoulder, wrist and hand). These could occur after stroke and require prompt treatment to prevent further disability.

Once you have defined your problems, you can make your plans. You will be set your goals with your physician or nurse. You can measure the degree to which you are meeting these goals and what might have worked for you to enable you to do so. Keeping a record in this way can help you to continue to meet your goal of staying healthy and living a quality life.

This chapter has a list of possible health problems. Within each of the sub-chapters that relate to your needs, there are three parts: Part One gives you information about the problem, Part Two gives you information about what could work to solve the problem, and Part Three is a planning sheet that can serve as your own log or record. Once you have identified the problem on the planning sheet, you can then set goals along with your nurse or doctor. As you keep your own record, you can learn more and more what changes to make either in medication with your physician's advice or life style. You will establish what works for you. You can also see how well you are doing. Keeping a record can help you to stay healthy long after you leave the hospital.

URINE MANAGEMENT

What is the Problem?

When someone experiences a stroke, he or she frequently has trouble staying dry or difficulty emptying the bladder that can result in an infection. Stroke can also affect one's ability to recognize when it is time to urinate, or the ability to call for assistance if recognition is present. Additionally the weakness in one's leg/arm affect the person's ability to get to the bathroom independently. If someone has had prior difficulty with dribbling or frequent nighttime urination, that condition will make the difficulties resulting from the stroke even worse.

The reason for trouble in managing urination after a stroke depends on the way the nervous system works to control urination. Both halves of the brain normally contribute to managing the control of the bladder and the urine it holds. Bladder function can and usually does return after a stroke. Loss of usual control comes about when the connection between the upper brain (cortical) centers and the spinal cord and the bladder center are disrupted. Since the stroke affects the brain, the tendency is loss of awareness of control and results in emptying at an inappropriate time. There may also be retention of urine because the muscle emptying the bladder does not act in a coordinated fashion to empty itself.

The problem is in control of the urinary bladder rather than in the kidneys where the urine is made. The kidneys automatically cleanse the blood of waste products that travel in liquid form down two pipes, called ureters, to the bladder. The bladder is where the urine is stored. When the bladder contracts, the urine moves into a narrow pipe that conducts it outside the body. Tiny valve-like muscles called sphincters open and close to control the urine flow. When the sphincters (internal and external) are closed, the urine is held in the bladder. There is another muscle called the detrusor across the top of the bladder. When this detrusor muscle is stretched and indicates the bladder is full, messages are sent to the brain suggesting urination. That muscle then contracts to empty the bladder in coordination with opening of the sphincters. Because both halves of the brain normally contribute to managing bladder control with the urine in it, bladder function can and frequently does return after a stroke.

"Incontinence" is uncontrolled emptying of urine at an unplanned time or location. Wetting oneself is not only embarrassing but can cause breakdown of the skin. Urinary retention occurs when the bladder holds too much urine and becomes overstretched. Dribbling of urine can then occur due to overflow from increased pressure. If there continues to be a buildup of urine in the bladder, the increased pressure can force the urine back up into the ureters and kidneys. When the bladder is not emptied, the stagnant urine can be a medium for bacterial infection. Overstretching can cause very tiny tears in the inside layers of the bladder wall and create potential sites for bacteria to grow. The goal in maintaining bladder health is recognizing and preventing infection, while at the same time emptying the bladder and protecting the skin.

The urinary problems caused by the stroke will be different depending on the person. For example, retention of urine in the bladder is a particular problem in males where an enlarged prostate can further complicate the situation caused by the stroke. The prostate, part of the reproductive system, is found just below the bladder and completely surrounds the outlet to the outside. Normally this causes no problem. But if the gland is enlarged, it constricts outflow of urine. The sphincter in the male is also fairly strong and can go into spasm and make emptying more difficult. After a stroke, the weak bladder muscle (the detrusor) has additional difficulty pushing the urine out of the urethra past the constriction caused by the enlarged prostrate gland. This difficulty results in urinary retention and can cause a bladder infection from the urine left behind.

Trouble with standing or sitting caused by the stroke presents additional problems. Normal bladder emptying is done in an upright position and creates an increase in intra-abdominal pressure aiding in the flow of urine from the bladder. Trying to empty the bladder into a bedpan or urinal while lying in bed also is less effective than sitting on a commode for women or standing for men. Becoming able to transfer from the bed to a commode can help to increase emptying.

When a person first goes to the hospital, a catheter is used to empty the bladder during the first few days after the stroke. During the time that fluids are given intravenously, there is need to ensure that the bladder is emptied. The use of an indwelling catheter for this purpose is common, yet likely to lead to infection because it provides a constant path for bacteria to get in the bladder. There is also the need to protect the skin against wetting and possible breakdown so that incontinence needs to be dealt with.

Another method is to empty the bladder with an "intermittent catheter." Intermittent catheterization is the timed (4-6 times a day) use of a catheter to drain the bladder of urine that is present, with removal of the catheter after draining. However, incontinence can occur between intermittent catheterizations and cause skin irritation and break down. With these competing goals, an indwelling catheter is usually the choice in acute-care hospitals. Unfortunately this may result in infection.

Upon arriving at the rehabilitation setting, the indwelling catheter is generally removed in order to reduce the chances of infection. One of three events can follow: 1) the person is continent of urine, has the sensation to urinate, and the ability to hold it until reaching the toilet; 2) the person is incontinent of urine and has difficulty holding the urine when the sensation to void does occur, or 3) the person is not aware of the sensation to urinate, but has some 'dribbling' along with urinary retention. Retention is confirmed by doing a 'bladder scan' by ultrasound to measure the amount of urine present. Another way of checking retention is to put a catheter in to check the volume of urine present after voiding. If the volume is greater than 150 cc on three trials, it is treated as retention. This is called post-voiding residual (PVR). The goal is to prevent over-distention and cause adequate emptying so that infection does not have a chance to multiply until urinary control can be re-established.

There is need to find out whether an infection is present that can contribute to the difficulty in urination. Once the infection is cleared up, many of the problems go away. Infections can be treated with the appropriate antibiotic. Table 5.1 describes some of the signals you can use to tell your doctor if you think you may have an infection. Looking at the urine under a microscope can help confirm that an infection is present right away. One looks for white blood cells which reflect the presence of infection. Finding out the particular bacteria causing the infection and their sensitivity to one or another antibiotic can take 48 hours, but one can start treatment immediately and change the medication if necessary.

Table 5.1 Symptoms of Urinary Infection

- burning with urination (dysuria)
- an increased need to urinate (frequency)
- difficulty starting a stream (hesitancy)
- a sense of incomplete emptying after voiding (fullness)
- difficulty holding the urine (urgency)
- a change in urine color, clarity, or odor
- fever, chills, or back pain
- increased or new episodes of urinary incontinence

What Works

Drinking at least a quart of water can help flush out the kidneys and bladder. Drinking water also helps to dilute any bacteria that tend to be present. When the amount of bacteria multiply to a particular level (greater than 100,000 per ml), illness and infection are far more likely. If the problem is not due to infection; or persists after the infection is properly treated, then the action of the bladder (weak detrusor or enlarged bladder) may need to be modified. There are several different kinds of medication that can be used. Table 5.2 describes the kinds of medication used for the various problems.

What works depends on figuring out what is wrong. One female with a recent stroke shows the problem with retention. She found herself having to urinate very often and never felt that she could empty her bladder completely. She did not have an infection when her urine was examined. When checked by inserting a catheter into her bladder, there was about 200 cc of urine that remained. Her post-voiding residual (PVR) was excessive. The problem apparently was due to her bladder muscle not contracting as well as before her stroke. She was started on a medicine (bethanechol) that caused her

Table 5.2 Treatment for Urinary Problems

- If infection is present, use antibiotics and large amount of fluid.
- If retention is present in men, use drugs to relax sphincter with enlarged prostate (e.g., Terazosin).
- If incomplete emptying and retention is present in women, use drugs to increase the strength of contraction of the bladder (e.g., Bethanechol).
- If there is complete emptying, but urgency and frequency and no infection, use drugs to reduce the contraction (irritation) of the bladder (e.g., Oxybutynin).

bladder to contract more forcefully. With the use of medication, she was able to empty her bladder more completely. She no longer needed to urinate as often and her PVR was less than 150 cc. Thus the need for intermittent catheterization was eliminated.

A man who had an enlarged prostrate had been getting up several times a night to urinate before his stroke. After the stroke, he was unable to get up to urinate without assistance since he had a weak leg. He was no longer able to empty his bladder, even though a urinal was available to him in his bed. He was given a medicine to relax his urinary sphincter, and he was then able to empty his bladder.

One woman has had to urinate frequently during the night for many years. She had been doing so without difficulty and had put up with the annoyance. However, once she had weakness of the leg associated with her stroke, she could no longer get up on her own at the need to do so. She found herself wet at night. Getting stronger and becoming able to do a safe transfer enabled her to regain continence.

A man with a recent stroke was incontinent of urine. Because of his skin being wet, sores began to form on the skin. Wearing a diaper caused a rash. He had difficulty in speaking because of his stroke but also did not seem to be aware of when he needed to urinate. There could be several things that could be done, but it was necessary to determine first whether he had any infection or retention. His urine tested okay, and there was no infection. He did have some urine still present after he had emptied his bladder. We could deal with the retention by giving him a medication (Terazosin) that helped open the sphincter. You remember that in men, there is a fairly strong sphincter than can also be closed off by an enlarged prostate. This medication enabled him to empty his bladder more fully. However, he was still incontinent. When his wife was present, she was able to read his signals that he needed to urinate. She was accustomed to his signals and able to get him to stay dry by giving him a urinal. When it was not possible to get him to a toilet when leaving the house; for example, he was able to wear a condom-type external catheter to protect his skin.

Alternatively, a toileting schedule every 2-3 hours can be used to help re-train the bladder. This increases the person's awareness of the need to urinate and protects against the bladder becoming too full. It also permits the person to stay dry and avoid skin breakdowns. Pelvic floor exercises have been useful in helping to correct simple incontinence.

When intermittent catheterization and medication are not effective, further testing by a urologist may be necessary. Tests performed by the urologist are "urodynamics" and require special catheters. During these tests, the bladder walls can be checked to find tears, masses, or inflammation. Fluid can be put in the bladder to: 1) determine how much the bladder will hold before the person is aware of the sensation to urinate, 2) how much pressure it takes from the full bladder for it to open, 3) how much stretch the detrusor will take before it responds and contracts, and 4) if the contraction of the detrusor is coordinated with the opening of the sphincters. Lastly, it can determine if the contraction is strong enough to empty the bladder. Based on these findings, the urologist makes recommendations.

There was a woman who had a stroke affecting the strength in her left side and making it difficult to transfer to a toilet without assistance. She had problems emptying her bladder and had retained volumes averaging 150 - 250 cc when placed on a bedpan. She therefore required routine intermittent catheterization. She rarely had the sensation of the need to urinate and also suffered from incontinence. Initial treatment consisted of intermittent catheterization and a toileting schedule. Her retained-urine volumes remained high in spite of this, so the evaluation by a urologist was sought. In her case she was found to have enough strength in her detrusor coordinated with opening of the sphincter to not need medication. Intermittent catheterization was stopped and a Foley catheter was placed because it was found that her uterus (womb) was pressing on her bladder and caused obstruction of urine outflow.

Making your own plan involves keeping a record of your urine in comparison to your goal for adequate emptying of your bladder or alleviating symptoms of infection. You should also track any medication or other actions you are taking to achieve your goal.

Exercise 5.1 Making a Plan for Myself

1. What is the problem?

The first decision is whether a problem exists. We can then determine the cause of the problem and help alleviate it. The purpose of the bladder is to store urine so that one can empty the bladder at the appropriate time and place without undue inconvenience. There can be problems in lack of control of the bladder (incontinence). Some people also complain of having to go more often (frequency) and having to go right away (urgency) as signal of infection. Less commonly there may be pain on urination associated with each of the above.

- incontinence _____
- frequency _____
- urgency _____
- other _____

This exercise gives you a chance to score yourself on this item. You can place the date for your "status" at the level where you are now. "Goal" is the level you would like to be at the next time you evaluate yourself along with your nurse or doctor. The next date may be one week or one month or whatever you and your doctor or nurse decide. Early during your treatment after having had a stroke, more frequent checks are done. Later on you may wish to wait longer. At the end of each time you can once again measure your new status and compare it to your goal. You can also see what worked to bring about the change and how much you have contributed to answering these questions.

2. Following my plan

Participation: Agreement (A) Confirmed Agreement (CA) Statement (S) Specific Statement (SS)			
Date	**Status/Progress**	**Goals**	**What Works**
	☐	☐	☐
	☐	☐	☐

BOWEL MANAGEMENT
What is the Problem?

The first decision that needs to be made is that a problem exists. The problem could be constipation with resultant discomfort or loss of control. As in the case of urination, where dribbling can occur because of lack of emptying, loss of bowel control can frequently be an outgrowth of constipation. After a stroke, it is common for the person's normal bowel habits to be disrupted. There is a change in diet and reduction in amount of exercise and general activity. Just as with emptying the bladder, not being able to sit up while trying to move one's bowels also contributes to disruption.

Understanding how the bowels work can help you to understand what has gone wrong and how you can contribute to fixing it. The gastrointestinal tract is the system from which the body receives its nutrition. It is a long tube from the mouth through the esophagus, stomach, small intestines, large intestines, and rectum. Food stimulates rhythmic waves called peristalsis which moves the food through the stomach where it is digested and finally moves into the small intestines. The food components are absorbed through the walls into the blood stream. The waste that remains behind forms a bulk and causes a stretch of the intestinal walls. The stretch causes a stimulus to occur that results in peristalsis, or movement of the bulk of the waste forward into the large intestine.

The large intestines (colon) are made up of three sections found in an inverted 'u-shape' and named by their placement in the abdomen. The three sections are called the ascending, transverse and descending colon. The last is the portion closest to the rectum and outlet. It is in the ascending colon where the waste products of digestion are collected in a liquid form initially. As the waste moves through the colon, water is reabsorbed resulting in a more solid form ready for elimination. This solid form is called feces and collects in the last part of the intestines called the rectum. The rectum serves as a storage place like the bladder for urine.

When the rectum fills with the bulk of waste, it causes a stretch there. The nerves in the rectum sense the stretch and send messages to the brain indicating time for elimination. The rectal sphincter helps hold the feces in the rectum until we reach the bathroom. Learned control of this elimination is stored in the frontal lobe of our brains.

After a stroke, there can be a breakdown in the communication between the intestines, rectum, and the brain that interferes with satisfactory elimination. There may be a loss of sensation or decreased awareness of fullness in the bowels, rectum, and muscles of the area. The loss causes decreased urge and delay in elimination. There may be bowel incontinence associated with a sudden urge or spontaneous evacuation without any prior signal. Bowel problems after a stroke are usually a result of immobility, decreased fluid intake, or inadequate fiber intake. One may not have moved the bowels on the usual schedule because of problems in getting out of bed. Drugs can have side effects that cause constipation; e.g., antacids, narcotic analgesics, and diuretics.

The problems frequently seen are constipation and/or incontinence. Constipation is defined as the infrequent or difficult elimination of stool/feces. Any change from normal bowel habits person is identified as a problem. In general, when the feces stay in the intestines too long (more than three days), the fluid that helps it remain bulky is reabsorbed and causes difficulty in its passage. Problems related to constipation include impaction, diarrhea, and skin breakdown due to incontinence. If the feces becomes too hard, it can become impacted and block the passage of formed stool. When this occurs, liquid stools leak out around the blockage. This incontinence must be evaluated for correct treatment. An impaction may require an enema or more aggressive treatment such as manual removal. When constipation is frequent or becomes chronic, the walls of the rectum become over stretched and lose the sense of stretch triggering the urge to defecate. The goal in maintaining bowel health is recognizing and preventing constipation while at the same time having regular bowel movements without incontinence.

What Works?

After dealing with any impaction, treatment of constipation includes increasing bulk of the feces by a high fiber diet. See Table 5.3 for some common foods and their fiber content. In addition, fiber can come from sources other than one's diet. These bulk formers go under different names. The total amount of fiber in your diet or with bulk former can vary. Most people do well with 20 gms/day, but some

Table 5.3 High Fiber Foods

Food	Amount	Grams of dietary fiber
Breads and cereals		
All-Bran	⅔ cup	17.0
Bran Buds	⅔ cup	15.8
Bran Flakes	¾ cup	4.0
Grape Nuts	½ cup	2.8
Oatmeal	¾ cup	1.6
Shredded Wheat	1 biscuit	2.2
Whole wheat bread	1 slice	2.1
Bran muffin	1 medium	3.5
Fruits		
Apple, raw with skin	1 medium	2.8
Applesauce	½ cup	1.4
Apricots, raw	3 medium	1.4
Banana, raw	1 medium	1.6
Blackberries, raw	1 cup	3.3
Orange	1 medium	2.8
Pear, raw	1 medium	4.1
Pear, canned	½ cup	1.2
Prunes, dried	4	5.4
Prune juice	1 cup	2.5
Strawberries, raw	1 cup	2.8
Vegetables		
Asparagus	½ cup	1.5
Avocado, raw	½ medium	2.3
Beans, green	¼ cup	2.0
Broccoli, cooked	⅔ cup	4.1
Brussels sprouts, cooked	6.8 medium	2.9
Cabbage, raw	½ cup	1.7
Carrots, raw	1 large	2.9
Carrots, cooked	⅔ cup	3.1
Cauliflower, raw	½ cup	1.0
Cauliflower, cooked	½ cup	1.1
Celery, raw	1 stalk	1.8
Corn on the cob	4-inch ear	4.7
Lettuce	3½ ounces	1.5
Mushrooms	10 small	1.2
Peas, green, canned	⅔ cup	6.3
Spinach, cooked	½ cup	6.3
Tomato, raw	1 small	1.5
Other		
Ryekrisp	2 triple crackers	1.6
Wheat snacks	15	1.1

Table 5.4 Sample Plan

Participation: Agreement (A)	Confirmed Agreement (CA)	Statement (S)	Specific Statement (SS)
Date	**Status/Progress**	**Goals**	**What Works**
8/12	☐ Bowel movement every few days at no established time	☐	☐
8/14	☐ Met goal	☐ B.M. every day in the morning	☐ 2 tabs Senakot night before
8/16	☐ Met goal	☐ Maintain schedule	☐ 1 tab Senakot; increase fiber by selecting more fruits and vegetables on menu to 15 gms
8/18	☐ Met goal	☐ Maintain schedule	☐ No Senakot; oatmeal, fruit
8/18	☐	☐ Maintain schedule	☐

people need more. Fluids and water up to 2-3 liters per day are necessary since the fiber holds water to provide the bulk in the stool encouraging peristalsis. Exercise/ activity improves abdominal muscle strength and enables persons to bear down to empty the rectum. As before the stroke, it is important to get back on a convenient schedule for elimination. This could be after meals since eating does stimulate the action of the colon.

There are many over-the-counter medications that one may use. It is important, however, to understand the action of each choice and not over-medicate with them; e.g., stool softeners, stimulants to increase peristalsis, and suppositories or enemas. The important point is to start by getting cleaned out and then get on a regular schedule consistent with your normal pattern. This could be daily, every other day,

Exercise 5.2 Making a Plan for Myself

1. What are my problems?

- incontinence   _____
- constipation   _____
- abdominal discomfort   _____

Remember these problems may not be due to the stroke alone. Many people have different patterns of bowel elimination. The effect of the stroke can vary with the person.

This exercise gives you a chance to score yourself on this item. You can place the date for your "status" at the level where you are now. "Goal" is the level you would like to be at the next time you evaluate yourself along with your nurse or doctor. The next date may be one week or one month or whatever you and your doctor or nurse decide. Early during your treatment after having had a stroke, more frequent checks are done. Later on you may wish to wait longer. At the end of each time you can once again measure your new status and compare it to your goal. You can also see what worked to bring about the change and how much you have contributed to answering these questions.

2. Following my plan

Participation: Agreement (A) Confirmed Agreement (CA) Statement (S) Specific Statement (SS)			
Date	**Status/Progress**	**Goals**	**What Works**
	☐	☐	☐
	☐	☐	☐
	☐	☐	☐

or every three days. Every person has his/her own time for having a bowel movement. It is also important for you to help set the time for you to get back on your own schedule.

Making your own plan involves keeping a record of your bowel elimination in comparison to your goal and track any medication, diet, or your other actions to achieve your goal. Table 5.4 illustrates a log kept by a woman with a recent stroke. She found that her previous problems with irregular bowels had become worse now that she spent much more time in bed and she felt less control over the foods brought in. She also was receiving several different medications relating to her bowels as well as becoming more familiar with the fiber content of various foods. She was able to reduce the use of medication while increasing the fiber content of her diet and maintain her goal of regular bowel movement. She was able to state her goal and monitor results and soon stating what worked. These statements met the criterion of specificity by describing not only "what," but "when" and "how much" in terms of grams of fiber.

MAINTAINING NUTRITION

What is the Problem

Maintaining proper nutrition requires the ability to eat the right amount of food, chew and swallow it, and have the food absorbed by the stomach and small intestines for the body to use. This can be affected by appetite, dentures, cavities, food appearance and taste, as well as the ability of the person to be able to feed him/herself. All these can be problems for persons with a recent stroke. Particularly important is the ability to swallow without the food and/or liquids going into the lungs. Food going into the lungs is called aspiration. This sub-chapter deals with the problems of maintaining adequate nutrition when there is a problem affecting the normal intake of food.

The body needs food to maintain itself and meet the energy(calorie) requirements of daily activity. The amount of nutrition needed is based on a person's height, weight, activity level and disease/ illness process. One can be overweight but malnourished. Those that have been drinking alcohol consistently may also be malnourished. The presence of skin ulcers, fever, nausea with vomiting and or diarrhea may require higher calories and additional vitamins such as Vitamin C and zinc to assist in the repair of the wound/healing process.

Many people with stroke have problems with adequate nutrition even before their stroke. They may not eat enough while in the hospital right after the stroke. Blood tests such as protein, albumin, or pre-albumin are indicators of nutritional status. Additional blood tests such as BUN/creatinine, sodium (Na+), potassium (K+), and cholesterol profiles can guide the physician or Nurse Practitioner in making dietary recommendations. Occasionally, the need to take a particular kind of medicine such as Coumadin (Warfarin), a blood thinner, may influence the diet order to be Vitamin K controlled as discussed in Chapter 6. Diet changes can contribute to reducing the chances of having a recurrent stroke. Therefore, we start by limiting the amount of salt (4 gms) and cholesterol (0.3 gms) in your hospital diet. This is called the American Heart Association (AHA) heart-healthy diet as discussed in Chapter 6 and is based on the fact that many persons who have had a stroke have high blood pressure and/or elevated cholesterol. Persons with diabetes need to follow a diet with a restriction in the numbers of calories and the percentage of calories that come from sugars/carbohydrates. If a person has kidney problems, the physician may also restrict foods high in potassium (K+) and protein.

An adequate amount of water and other fluids (1-3 liters/quarts each day) is essential. This is also based on the medical issues, activity level, problems with constipation or diarrhea. Of course, the more you drink, the concern for needing help to get to the bathroom to pass urine can be a concern. A certain amount of liquids is necessary to prevent bladder infections (see earlier discussion on urine management). Problems with constipation may require increased fluids, increased activity, and increase in fiber intake, and occasionally the use of medications (see earlier discussion on bowel management).

The kind of diet as mentioned above is based on the food contents. The calories come from the amount of energy it takes a body to burn off the food it has consumed. Each kind of nutrient, carbohydrates (sugars), proteins and fats, provide a different amount of calories for the body to break them down to be used by the cells. Carbohydrates are the sugars for the body. Diabetics have trouble using the sugars because they don't have enough insulin to help break it down. For this reason diabetics take medicines that help prevent too much sugar from being in their blood. Proteins such as that found in meat and dairy products provide energy for the cells as well as provide building blocks for repairing the body. Fats provide even moreenergy than the other nutrients. If they are not used by the cells right away, they are the easiest to store away. For example, a gram of fat provides 9 calories when it is burned, but carbohydrates and proteins provide 4 calories per gram. There are about 4-5 grams in a teaspoon; about 15 grams in a tablespoon; about 30 grams in an ounce. The total number of calories can be measured by the number of grams times the number of calories in each gram.

If the ability to swallow is not safe, and the lungs are not protected by the cough response, one can get pneumonia from the food getting into the lungs. Prevention of aspiration while maintaining nutrition is the goal. Occasionally, the swallowing mechanism is too weak and a feeding tube may be needed to bypass the normal swallowing mechanism. The tubes can also be used to give the necessary medications and water as well as other nutrients. It is important to recognize that certain long-acting medications cannot be crushed and used in tubes. See Chapter 7 for an in-depth discussion of "dysphagia" or the swallowing problem that may occur after a stroke.

There are two kinds of tubes that you may see. One type is inserted into the nose and is called a naso-gastric (NG) tube. It goes down the throat into the stomach. This tube is usually used when the problem is likely to be temporary (about 3-4 weeks or less). The position of this tube is important. If it is pulled out from where it has been placed, the tube feeding might go into the lungs.

If it is not likely that the person will be safe when swallowing after several weeks, a swallowing test called a Modified Barium Swallowing test (MBS) may be recommended. It is done by the speech-language pathologist and the radiologist to determine if a change in texture or posture would be helpful of if there is a likelihood that aspiration would continue to occur. If the latter is the case, the doctor may recommend placement of a stomach tube called a PEG (percutaneous endoscopic gastrostomy tube). This tube goes directly from the skin of the belly into the stomach and bypasses the throat so that there is less discomfort. The PEG is put in by a gastroenterologist under sterile conditions. The need for a tube is not usually permanent, and once

Table 5.5 Content of Supplemental Diet

PRODUCT	Jevity®	Ensure Plus®	Glucerna®	Nepro®
Calories/cc	1.06	1.5	1.0	2.0
Protein g/Liter (1%)	44.3 (16.7)	54.9 (14.7)	41.8 (16.7)	69.9 (14.0)
CHO g/Liter (%)	154.4 (54.3)	200.0 (53.3)	95.8 (34.3)	215.2 (43.0)
Fat g/Liter (%)	34.7 (20.0)	53.3 (32.0)	54.4 (49.0)	95.6 (43.0)

the swallowing is documented to be safe, it can be easily removed by the gastroenterologist.

Ongoing evaluation and exercises will be done by the speech-language pathologist until such time as the tube can be removed.

Once decided which method (by mouth or tube) of nutrition will be prescribed, the correct diet will be ordered. Liquid nutrition may be started in order to prevent malnutrition. There are many types of liquid nutrition available depending on the person's medical problems. Some liquids provide a higher fiber content to ensure satisfactory bowel movements. Others are specifically designed for diabetics with a lower sugar content. Still others are available with low potassium and protein for those persons with kidney problems. Some have higher amount of calories in the same size can (240 cc) to allow more calories in a smaller volume of fluid. All liquid nutrition cans have 70-80% free water in them. The contents are listed on each can. One can use a blender to use your own foods to make the liquid diet. The prepared liquid diets, however, are obviously more convenient. Table 5.5 lists the contents of many of the diets. The adequacy of the feedings can be measured by repeating the blood tests mentioned earlier in this section, by maintenance of body weight, and by maintaining satisfactory bowel and bladder function.

What Works

Occasionally, the person is discharged while still needing tube feedings. When that is the case, it is important that the patient understand as well as the family care giver how to manage the tube and the pump machines and/or the syringes used to introduce the diet into the tube. The patient usually has difficulty with only one functioning hand. Home-care nurses can also help after there has been training while the patient is still in the hospital. One also needs to watch out for infection as long as the tube is in place.

The following illustrates some of the things one can do to overcome nutritional problems. A man with diabetes and also on dialysis had to have a triple-by-pass heart surgery. During the surgery, he had a stroke and was left paralyzed on his left side. He had occasional coughing when he ate and drank liquids. There was concern that he would aspirate. A swallowing study was done that showed food going into the lungs. It was recommended that a PEG be placed until such time that his swallow was strong enough to protect his lungs.

It was recommended by the dietitian that his daily caloric intake be near 2200 calories/day because of his size and level of activity as well as his being on dialysis. It took at least nine cans/day of Glucerna (especially for diabetics) to meet the required number of calories. (Each can contains 240 calories, and 9 cans provide about 2200 calories). He took six of those cans through the night, while hooked up to the machine that pumped the tube feeding in continuously at about 120 cc/hour. (This took about 12 hours). The additional three cans were divided up throughout the day at meal times when each took about 2 hours. It became apparent that the patient was scheduled to be "tied up" to the feeding tube machine for 18 hours each day. This was unacceptable because it interfered with things he needed to do in therapy. In order to deal with this time-consuming task, he cut back on the amount of (calories) he would agree to take. This resulted in about 1500 calories each day. He began to lose weight. It then became obvious that he was not receiving the nutrition he needed. The goal was to maintain nutrition without aspiration.

There was another way he could get the needed nutrition in a shorter period of time. Nepro, a special formula for persons on dialysis with higher calories in a smaller volume (480 calories per can) would need only five cans/day. (This could take a total of 10 hours per day, some of which would be while he was asleep.) He received a sufficient amount of fluid despite the more concentrated feedings. The five cans gave him 1200 cc and it was supplemented by a water flush to clear the tube of about 100 cc at the end of the feedings. He would also get some fluid to flush any of his medications. Eventually, his swallowing was stronger, documented by another MBS. Then the PEG was removed by the gastroenterologist after the patient was able to eat 3/4 of each meal three times/day Once the tube was removed, the goal was to maintain nutrition compatible with his medical needs and give him the ability to choose foods he liked.

Answers to some concerns expressed by his care givers included: Will the tube be uncomfortable? The presence of the tube should not cause any discomfort unless it is pulled on, such as when changing positions during the continuous feedings. There should be no discomfort during the feeding unless too much air gets in the tube, or unless the feeding or water flush is too cold and causes some cramping.

If the volume is more than the person is used to, it may be uncomfortable for a short while. One can usually tolerate a 240 cc of 'one shot' (bolus) feeding followed by 50 - 100 cc of water flush. Some medications go into the tube better if given in the water. Still other medications flow in better in the weight of the feeding. If the feeding spills or comes apart from the tube, it easily washes up. Once the tube is used several times, the plug on the end becomes loose. Then one may need to tape the plug in during feedings or in between feedings.

Some questions patients ask about the use of tube include:

- How much give and how much resistance should I feel? Very little resistance should be felt and you should actually be able to see the feeding flow fairly freely. If it is necessary to push food or medications through, then it may need more follow-up flushing to wash it out. Medications, however, may be a bit more sluggish.
- What do I do to care for the tube? The person with the tube should be able to take a shower even with the tube in. Gently wash the site with soap and warm water and blot dry afterwards. Sometimes there would need to be an antibiotic ointment applied in small amounts around the tube. When caring for the tube, you must watch the site for any signs of infection, including, redness, swelling, warmth , new drainage, new color of drainage, and/or tenderness. The doctor needs to be informed immediately if infection is suspected.
- What happens if the tube gets clogged? Flush the tube with warm water first. If this is unsuccessful, use a cola drink that has fizz in it, and let the visiting nurse know, so she may inspect it.

Exercise 5.3 Making a Plan for Myself

1. What is the problem?

- Calories I Need   _____
- Water I Need   _____
- Fiber I Need   _____
- Special Diet Limitations (sugar, protein, fat, etc.) _____

This exercise gives you a chance to score yourself on this item. You can place the date for your "status" at the level where you are now. "Goal" is the level you would like to be at the next time you evaluate yourself along with your nurse or doctor. The next date may be one week or four weeks or whatever you and your doctor or nurse decide. At the end of each time you can once again measure your new status and compare it to your goal. You can also see what worked to bring about the change and how much you have contributed to answering these questions. We hope that you can answer these questions more and more on your own.

2. Following my plan

Participation: Agreement (A) Confirmed Agreement (CA) Statement (S) Specific Statement (SS)			
Date	**Status/Progress**	**Goals**	**What Works**
	☐	☐	☐
	☐	☐	☐
	☐	☐	☐
	☐	☐	☐

CENTRAL POST STROKE PAIN SYNDROME
What is the Problem

Pain is a common complaint following a stroke. There are several different kinds of pain. Frequently a patient may experience more than one type of pain. In this section we will be talking about what is called "central" pain. That means that is caused by something that happened inside the brain. Pain is something that people have had in their lives but is usually related to an injury that you can understand, like a cut or a broken bone. The pain then comes on suddenly. This pain is different and comes on in the part of the body that may have been affected by the stroke. But the pain may not come on right away. It may take as long as several months for it to appear. By then, most people would not necessarily connect its appearance with the stroke. Yet it is directly related to the stroke. If you develop pain on your involved side, you should discuss it with your physician for evaluation for possible post-stroke pain syndrome and treatment options, considering your other medical problems.

Post-stroke pain can vary. The pain is mostly burning in character but could be aching, sharp, or stabbing and in rare cases itching. Pain can be mild, moderate or severe, constant or come and go, and can interfere with sleep. Non-painful stimuli, such as touch, can be unpleasant and perceived as pain. Emotional stress, cold, and movement can increase pain. The pain is on part or whole involved side (face, arm, leg, and — very infrequently — trunk). Nearly all persons with stroke afflicted with post-stroke pain have trouble feeling a sharp pin or feeling warm or cold on the skin.

This helps to explain why this pain comes on and why it might be delayed in coming on. The present theory suggests that this type of pain is related to damage to the connection between the skin and the brain which carries these messages. When the normal messages do not reach the brain, other abnormal messages which may feel like pain take their place.

What Works

One of the most important things about pain is that it can be affected by other sensations or feelings. It can be modified. But one thing important to understand is that at times it cannot be totally eliminated.

Then the goal becomes not to let the pain run your life. A psychologist can assist you with this matter. See Chapter 9 for an in-depth discussion of pain-management strategies. Reassuring patients that the pain does not indicate damage or injury will decrease their anxiety about the pain. For some patients with mild pain, reassurance is sufficient, and these patients may choose not to have any further treatment. There are ways to increase one's ability to tolerate the strange feelings when you are touched. It is often helpful when stretching to make the movements "smooth with no jerky movements." Transcutaneous Electrical Nerve Stimulation (TENS) is the name for a technique that can be helpful. Your physical therapist can teach you how to use TENS.

Narcotics and most analgesics and nonsteroidal anti-inflammatory drugs, such as Aspirin and Ibuprofen, are not effective in treatment of post-stroke pain syndrome. Most effective medications are "tricyclic" antidepressants (such as Amitriptyline) and can relieve pain in up to 75% of patients. But pain relief may not occur right away. It generally starts in about one week after beginning treatment. Pain intensity may fluctuate, and improvement may consist of longer periods of less severe pain. Improvement may also be shown by a shrinkage of the area in which pain is felt. If pain doesn't improve in two weeks, it may still respond with an increase in the amount of medication. All these drugs cause dryness of mouth. This can be overcome by using chewing gum. This type of antidepressant medication works on this pain, not on any depression. You should know the drugs that are being prescribed for pain and not for their antidepressant effect. People vary in their response to these medications, in part because of the type of pain they are experiencing. There are several other medications that can be effective when added to "tricyclic" antidepressants, such as medications used to treat convulsions.

In one case, a woman with recent stroke resulting in mild left-sided weakness and difficulty in feeling a sharp pin, complained of pain in her left leg. Her left leg was very sensitive to touch and she was unable to put weight on it. She had to use a wheelchair. It helped her to understand that her pain was due to the stroke. She learned from a psychologist how to use relaxation techniques. She also started on "tricyclic" antidepressants (Elavil®). She learned from her physical therapist how to gradually desensitize her leg. Within 10 days, the patient's pain was decreased and she was able to bear weight on her left

Exercise 5.4 Making a Plan for Myself

1. What is the problem

   If you are diagnosed as having post-stroke pain , then making your own plan involves keeping a record of your pain and the activity you are able to carry out even if the pain persists at some level. The first decision is to identify what about the pain is most important. Then with treatment, you will be able to see your progress with decreasing pain. Your pain may not totally disappear, but could decrease in intensity and duration.

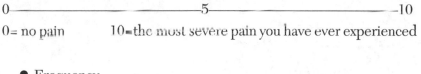

INTENSITY

0————————————————————————5————————————————————————-10

0= no pain   10=the most severe pain you have ever experienced

- Frequency
- Activity
- Duration

   This exercise gives you a chance to score yourself. You can place the date for your "status" at the level you are now. "Goal" is the level for pain relief you would like to achieve at the next time you evaluate yourself, along with your doctor. The next date may be from one to four weeks. You can again measure your new status and compare it to your goal. You can also see what worked to bring about the change. You can also consider how much you contributed to answering these questions.

   2. Following my plan

Participation: Agreement (A) Confirmed Agreement (CA) Statement (S) Specific Statement (SS)			
Date	**Status/Progress**	**Goals**	**What Works**
	☐	☐	☐

leg for transfers. She also began to learn how to walk. Because the patient's goal was to be able to walk, decreasing her pain made it possible for her to work with her therapist to accomplish that goal.

Post-stroke pain responds best to treatment when begun early. Your pain may not resolve entirely, but it might decrease in intensity and duration or vary on how often it comes (frequency).Even if the pain does not go away altogether, the relief may permit you to not let the pain run your life. The overall goal can be to carry on with your life and you can record the activities you were able to carry out. Medication may be required for a lifetime.

MUSCULOSKELETAL PAIN

What is the Problem

Pain in the affected shoulder and arm is a frequent complain of patients after having had a stroke. The pain tends to develop early, several weeks to several months after a stroke. It is especially common in persons who had severe weakness of the affected arm. The first cause of trouble with the shoulder is when weakness of the muscles affect the ability of the arm to remain in its socket. Because the shoulder muscles do not hold the arm in its proper place, injury is more likely when moving the arm of the person. "Subluxation" is the term used when the arm is not in its socket. The weight of the arm pulls it down out of the socket when the shoulder muscles that ordinarily keep it in place are too weak to hold it in. This is true early on after a stroke. When the arm is pulled, there can be injury to the nerves and other tissue around the arm. This can be one of the causes of pain that continues even later.

In the process of recovery after a stroke, the muscles tend to tighten up. This is called an increase in "tone" and can also cause pain, but for a different reason. The delicate coordinated rhythm of the shoulder blade (scapula) and the arm bone is lost. Connections between muscle and bones (tendons) get caught between the two bones when the arm moves. This is called "impingement."

Either way, there is limitation in the range of motion. The person has trouble not only with pain, but the pain is related to the range of motion. There may be pain after moving the arm through part of the full range. Each joint has what is called a normal range of motion. It is described in terms of the degrees through which the joint moves. The movement of the shoulder can be in different directions. One particularly important and frequently affected direction is lifting your arm away from your body (abduction). The normal range of motion for abduction is 180 degrees. Pain tends to occur when the arm is moved above 70 degrees. The goals are to get the movement to a functional range (100 degrees), to maintain function and at the same time to decrease the possibility of impingement.

Sometimes, pain may be present in the hand along with swelling of the hand, in addition to the pain in the shoulder. This is called the shoulder-hand syndrome. It is not entirely clear why, but there is increased activity of the nerves. The activity affects the blood vessels and other functions of the hand. There are different phases to this problem. The first is when there is swelling and warmth of the hand with increased sweating and tenderness of the joints of the hand. Later, there can be shiny, coolness of the skin. Even later there is stiffness of the joints with loss of range of motion.

What Works

Proper positioning of the arm and hand early on after the stroke is very important. When the arm muscles are loose, the arm should be supported when the persons is sitting. There are lap boards or an arm trough that may be used because of the stroke. After a stroke, there are persons who tend not to pay attention to the affected side. The patient may not realize that the arm is not in its proper place but is hanging down. Other people will need to remind the patient about this. There are many techniques that can be used for such reminders. When the patient is lying in bed or moved, the arm should not be pulled but protected. (See Chapter 8 for an in-depth discussion of arm positioning and care.)

The general principle of all treatments once a problem has occurred is to maintain functional range of motion. If swelling occurs in the hand, it seems useful to try to reduce the extent of such swelling. One way is to elevate the arm. There are also other techniques that the occupational therapist (OT) can show you how to massage the hand and to use specially designed elastic gloves to keep down the swelling once the massage has been useful. If the muscle tightness becomes so severe that stretching is not enough to maintain range of motion, there are other techniques that can be used. You can discuss them with your doctor. One new method is to use what is called "botulinum" injections. Once the muscles start to tighten up in the process of recovery, a "resting wrist and hand splint" at your wrist can help to keep the arm and hand in as functional a position as possible. This can help to prevent the hand and fingers from tightening up in a poor position ("contractures") that will make it harder to use the arm later on. The OT can help you with making a splint that will fit your hand. The OT will teach you and your family how to properly position your weak arm while you are lying and sitting.

Your therapist will also work with you to make it easier for there to be return of active movement at the shoulder. If the muscles have begun to tighten, there will be exercises for you and your family to help stretch the muscles and prevent limitation of range of motion. But it is not a good idea to use a pulley and weights to maintain range of motion. Your therapist can teach you and your family in the use of a heating pad or an ice pack to use for your shoulder. This should provide pain relief prior to doing your range of motion exercises. Sometimes it is useful to use medication to reduce the pain. This should also help you do the stretching exercises to improve the range of motion. Your physician can prescribe other medications or can inject your shoulder with cortisone-type medication. The important thing to realize is that you may get relief, and the problem is not usually permanent, although it can often be quite severe.

Judie Gray CRRN, MSN, Adult Nurse Practitioner, collaborated in writing Urine Management, Bowel Management and Maintaining Nutrition.

Exercise 5.5 Making a Plan for Myself

1. What is the problem

If you are diagnosed as having shoulder/hand pain with limitation of motion, then making your own plan involves keeping a record of your pain-free range of motion.

You can set your goal for a pain-free functional range of motion. Your physician/therapist can assist you with your range of motion measurement.

This exercise gives you a chance to record your range of motion. You can place the date of your status at the level you are now. Goal is the level pain free range of motion you would like to achieve at the next time you evaluate yourself, along with your doctor. The next date may be from one to four weeks. You can again measure your new status and compare it to your goal. You can also see what works to bring about the change. You can also consider how much you contributed to answering these questions.

2. Following my plan

Participation: Agreement (A) Confirmed Agreement (CA) Statement (S) Specific Statement (SS)			
Date	Status/Progress	Goals	What Works
	☐	☐	☐
	☐	☐	☐
	☐	☐	☐
	☐	☐	☐

6

Stroke Prevention

MARK N. OZER
FATEMEH MILANI

WHAT ARE THE PROBLEMS?

One major focus in staying healthy is to prevent another stroke. The same factor that caused the initial stroke may cause another. Disease affecting the blood vessels, whether in the heart or in the brain, is the major problem. Trouble with the blood vessels can also affect the legs and kidneys. Cardiac disease due to blockage of the blood vessels feeding the heart muscle is a major factor in the possibility of early death. Vascular disease affecting the heart can also lead to the formation of clots. These clots can travel to the brain and cause stroke.

The chance for stroke increases when certain risk factors are present. Some of these risk factors cannot be changed and are a part of our personal traits and medical history. These risk factors have to do with age, sex, race, and family inheritance. Persons at any age can have a stroke. However, the chances of having a stroke increase with age. Almost two-thirds of stroke occur in person over the age of 65. Males tend to have more strokes than females in their earlier years. This is believed to be related to the protection provided by female hormones, since after menopause the number of strokes in males is equal to females of the same age. Blacks tend to have more strokes than whites. The reason is not clear, but it is believed to be related to the incidence of high blood pressure in blacks and the different types of lifestyles and environment. Persons whose blood relatives have a history of heart disease or stroke are also at greater risk for a first or repeated stroke.

For the elderly male, or black, it becomes particularly important to try to do something about those controllable risk factors centered around lifestyle habits and treatable medical conditions. The major opportunities for preventing a stroke relate to high blood pressure and hardening of the arteries (a build-up of fatty deposits or "plaque" in the wall of the blood vessels). The life- style changes include modifying diet, exercising regularly, and stopping smoking. In all these situations, you can become a more active partner in affecting your future health. It is important that you find a physician who is going to work together with you in keeping you healthy. Smoking may contribute to both problems of high blood pressure and hardening of the arteries, as well as heart disease. Smoking tends to lower the "good" cholesterol (HDL) that helps to prevent plaque or fatty deposit build-up. Smoking can also cause certain blood cells, called platelets, to clump together and form blood clots cutting off the blood supply.

This chapter lists a number of possible risk factors that are treatable. Within these subchapters that relate to your needs, there are three parts. The first part gives you information about the problem, the second gives you information about what might work to solve the problem, and the third is a planning sheet that can serve as your log or record. Once you have identified the problem on that planning sheet, you can then set a goal along with your nurse or doctor. As you keep your own record, you can learn more and more about what effective changes you might make either in taking medication or in your lifestyle. You can also see how well you are doing. Keeping a record in this way can help you prevent another stroke once you leave the hospital.

USE OF BLOOD THINNERS

What is the Problem

Immobility occurring after a stroke can have even more serious consequences than causing problems with bladder and bowels. Still another consequence is the formation of blood clots in the legs which can go to the lungs cause problems with breathing.

The blood vessels form a system from the heart and then back. The farther away from the heart they are, the smaller they are. Arteries are the largest blood vessels that carry blood with oxygen from the heart and lungs to the farthest parts of the body. Arteries have a thin layer of muscle in the walls that helps the heart pump the blood. The blood carrying oxygen from the arteries then goes into the smallest vessels called capillaries. That is where the oxygen enters the cells to help the body to get the energy it needs. Returning blood from the cells carries waste from the cells toward the heart and then to the lungs to be cleaned and oxygen replaced. These blood vessels carrying waste products back to the heart are called veins. Blood flow through the veins depends on them being wide open with valves that prevent backflow and pumping action of the surrounding muscles.

After a stroke, the side of the body that is affected by the stroke has decreased movement. Therefore those muscles are not doing their job of helping pump the blood back towards the heart. This blood tends to sit around in the veins. The blood becomes thicker, has more blood clotting chemicals in it, and the lining of the veins are more likely to become inflamed. All of these factors can lead to clots forming. Persons with stroke are at great risk for clots to form during the first six weeks following their stroke due to this blood thickening tendency and less muscle action.

This standing clot is called a thrombosis. The most common places for the thrombus (clot) to form is in the affected leg. When it occurs in the deeper veins, it is called a deep vein thrombosis (DVT). When the thrombus blocks the normal return of blood, swelling occurs from a backup of extra fluid. That is why one watches for swelling in the leg as a possible result of the clot blocking the vein. There are other causes for swelling of the legs, but a clot is one of the causes to particularly watch for. If swelling of the leg is present, that may be a sign of blockage. At least half the time, there may be blockage of the vein but no sign of swelling. On the other hand, swelling may be present even though no blockage has actually occurred. For that reason, there are a number of tests used to check out whether blockage by clot is actually present. A sonar-type machine (called ultrasound) is used quite frequently today to check out the veins. Blood flowing throughout the veins will give a signal that can be measured. If there is no blood flow, there is no signal. Another sign is to press on the vein from the outside. Sonar outlines the blood vessels. If the vessel is open, then pressure from the outside can cause it to collapse. If it is blocked by clot, the vessel cannot be compressed.

The greatest danger of clot formation is when part of the clot will break off and go to the heart and then be pumped by the heart into the lungs. Clots in the veins of the thigh or the pelvis are more likely to break off than clots in the veins of the calf. These can be life threatening. The small clot that breaks off is called an embolism. If it goes to the lung, it is called a pulmonary embolism. If the clot in the blood vessels reaches the lung, that part of the lung is blocked off from oxygen entering the blood. There may not be enough oxygen to keep the person alive. Clots can go to the brain rather than into the lungs. A clot going to the brain can cause another stroke. If the heart beats irregularly or has weak walls, it does not move the blood out quickly enough to the lungs, brain, and body. Clots can develop in the heart. Clots can also occur in the presence of artificial heart valves. If the clot travels from the left side of the heart to the brain, a stroke can result. A clot traveling from the right side of the heart to the lungs causes difficulty with breathing as discussed earlier. Occasionally, someone will have a hole in the heart that allows some blood to cross through it from right to left and bypass the lungs. This does not usually cause a problem. However, if a person has a clot in a vein such as in the leg, that clot could pass through the hole and go to the brain and cause a stroke.

To better understand how these clots can occur, let's discuss how the heart works. The heart is divided into four chambers. The top two are called atria which receive blood and then pumps it to the bottom two chambers. These are called ventricles which pump blood out to the lung or the rest of the body. Both the atria and ventricles are divided into right and left sides. The right atrium of the heart receives blood from the veins in the body, empties it into the right ventricle which in turn pushes the blood to the lungs to receive oxygen. After the lungs have cleansed the blood, the blood returns to the left side of the heart through the left atrium. The blood is then emptied into the left ventricle and pushed out to the body and brain, full of oxygen and nutrients. Emptying and filling of the hearts chambers depends on delicate coordination of the beating heart. If a heart beats inefficiently as with irregular movements of the atria - called atrial fibrillation - or when the wall of the ventricle does not move properly, a clot may result. These are all potential problems treatable with drugs that cause blood to not clot as easily.

What Works

Prevention of thrombus formation in the leg veins works best when three methods are used. First, Heparin (a quick action blood thinner), lasts about 8-12 hours and is used to block normal clotting activity in the blood. Heparin is inactivated by stomach juices, and therefore cannot be taken by mouth. It is given twice a day, in a low dose by injection into the skin during both the acute medical and acute rehabilitation phases of hospitalization. Second, TEDS (elastic stockings that compensate for weak or paralyzed muscles by compressing the tissue around the veins to encourage fluid to go back to the heart) are used. It is for this reason that the stockings are tight, and it is important that they fit snugly without wrinkles. Third, exercise is part of treatment, and so it is helpful to start moving around as much as possible to use your leg muscles to stand and walk. Clots are much less frequent once you begin to move around.

If a blood clot does form in the legs, the treatment is to prevent it from breaking off and going to the lungs. We can quickly increase the thinning of the blood by increasing the dose of heparin by getting it into the blood intravenously (IV). Ultimately one can use a medicine (Warfarin/Coumadin) to be taken by mouth to thin the blood. It takes longer to work, but you can then continue it even after leaving the hospital. This medication needs to be monitored in terms of its effects. The management of the use of Warfarin will be discussed later in this chapter, when we consider other reasons to use it. The general recommendation is that treatment for DVT continue for about six months. If there is reason blood thinners cannot be used, a filter can be placed in the large vein that leads from the legs to the heart. This protects the lungs from the clot but does not reduce the likelihood of clot formation.

It is sometimes necessary to use blood thinners along with the filter. A recent case illustrates this situation. One man had a clot in his leg without any swelling. The clot was found when his leg was checked with sonar. Because his stroke was a result of hemorrhage into the brain, it was decided NOT to use blood thinners. A filter was placed in the large vein leading from the legs in order to prevent the clots from going to the lungs. The affected leg began to increase in size with the swelling due to increased blockage. It then became necessary to start the patient on blood thinners, along with the filter.

Warfarin is a blood thinner that slows the time it takes the blood to clot. We measure how "thin" the blood has become by what is called International Normalized Ratios (INR). It is very sensitive to some foods high in Vitamin K. Since there is already a Vitamin C, it is called Vitamin *K* to stand for *K*oagulability. Patients should avoid the foods that are particularly high in Vitamin K. See Table 6.1 for a list of foods to watch. If they are eaten just before their blood is checked, they will get a lower reading on their INR. This may lead the physician to increase the dosage of the Warfarin inappropriately resulting in an INR that is too high. There are also some medications that can interfere with effectiveness of the Warfarin. If a prescription drug is used, bring to the attention of your doctor that you are on Warfarin. Some common non-prescription drugs that can also interfere with the effects of Warfarin are the following:

- Aspirin
- Cold and cough medicines
- Laxatives
- Alcohol
- Vitamin E

Finally, today we now know that a number of herbs can also be implicated which is why it is important to keep your doctor informed about

Table 6.1 Food Interaction with Warfarin/(Coumadin)

It is important to maintain a consistent, balanced diet while on Warfarin. Inform your physician before making any significant change in your eating habits. In some cases, dietary changes may result in the need to adjust the dose of your anti-coagulant medicine. Look at the Vitamin K content listed for packaged foods.

Foods high in VITAMIN K can reduce the effects of your anticoagulant. Avoid significant changes in either increasing or decreasing your intake of these foods.

FOODS ESPECIALLY HIGH IN VITAMIN K:

VEGETABLES:	Asparagus, Brussels Sprouts, Broccoli, Cabbage, Chick Peas (garbanzo beans), Cauliflower, Kale, Lettuce, Spinach, Turnip Greens
OTHER:	Green Tea, Beef Liver, Apricot, Banana

Check with your physician before taking any Multivitamin or Nutritional Supplement containing Vitamin K.

what you are taking with Warfarin. Check with your doctor or pharmacist when you take *any* new medication so that your Warfarin dose can be adjusted or some other medication can be used. The effect of the Warfarin, therefore, must be measured on a regular basis by a blood test and reported to your doctor. Depending on the severity of the problem or potential problem, your doctor will set the INR range. For example, the INR range or goal might be 2.0-3.0. In other words, your blood would take 2 to 3 times longer to clot than normal blood. The higher the number, the longer it takes to clot, and the "thinner" your blood is. In this example, if your INR is less than 2, your blood is not thin enough. If it is higher than 3.5, it is too thin. This measurement must be checked regularly to ensure that there is enough of the medicine in your blood to be working effectively, but not too much to cause you harm. The frequency with which an INR is checked will vary with the patient and the problem leading to the use of Warfarin. This should be decided with your doctor.

If this is your first stroke, your doctor may recommend using an aspirin daily as a blood thinner. It is suggested that you use the kind that has a coating on it to protect your stomach. Ticlopidine HCL is a new blood thinner medication that has also been found to help prevent another stroke. It also has side-effects and must be monitored by a blood test when first started. It can interfere with the white blood cells your body needs to fight infection. If your "white count" goes below 3000 it should be discontinued. This should also be taken with food, as it can cause stomach irritation. Other drugs may also be used.

Bleeding is the thing to watch for. Bleeding in the urine is one common site. The urine will appear dark. Other signs of excessive blood thinning might be nosebleeds or blood in the stool. It may also take longer for your blood to clot if you cut yourself shaving. For this reason, an electric razor is recommended. It is helpful if you know the goal your doctor is using so you can do the things necessary to contribute to its effectiveness.

An example is a woman with a history of atrial fibrillation and disease of her heart valves after having had rheumatic fever as a child. She was on Warfarin (Coumadin) to protect against blood clots forming in the heart that might go to the brain. She had been on the same dose of Warfarin for several years. She had been seeing a doctor only rarely and did not have her INR checked. She was not aware of the proper INR range. She suddenly had right-sided weakness and trouble with language. Head CT showed a stroke caused by a clot. Her INR was 1.5 which was too low for persons with atrial fibrillation. She was not receiving a dose of the medication that was enough to protect her.

Another example is that of a 53-year-old man with numbness and tingling of his left arm. It cleared up after a few days. Head CT showed an injury to the brain on the right side. He was found to have a small hole in the wall separating the two receiving chambers of the heart. It was felt that a blood clot may have gone from his legs or pelvis to right side of the heart. Instead of being then pumped ordinarily to the lungs, the clot may have gone through the hole into the left-sided receiving chamber. The clot could then be pumped directly to the rest of the body, including the brain. If it went to the brain, the effects could be the brain injury that appeared on the head CT. To protect him against another stroke, he was started on Warfarin. He had recently moved to a new city and arranged to have his blood tested by a lab. The results of the test did not get back to the right person. Several months later, he awoke to find numbness in his entire right side and trouble both understanding and speaking. When he reached the hospital, his INR was 4.0 which was too high. This was far beyond the goal that had been sought for him. Head CT showed a hemorrhage in the left side of the brain.

Making your own plan involves keeping a record of your INR in comparison to your goal and keeping track of your medication as well as your other actions such as diet to control the thinning of your blood. Table 6.2 illustrates a case in which the person with stroke monitored his INR and the adjusted dose of Warfarin to meet the goal of 2.5-3.0.

HYPERTENSION MANAGEMENT

What is the Problem

High blood pressure or hypertension (HBP) is the number one risk factor for stroke. Hypertension can increase one's risk of stroke seven times more than in those with normal blood pressure. The higher the blood pressure, the greater the risk.

Table 6.2 Sample Plan To Monitor INR

Participation: Agreement (A) Confirmed Agreement (CA) Statement (S) Specific Statement (SS)			
Date	**Status/Progress**	**Goals**	**What Works**
8/30	☐ 3.3	☐	☐
9/02	☐ 2.6	☐ 2.5–3.0	☐ Hold Warfarin
9/05	☐ 3.0	☐ 2.5–3.0	☐ 2 mg Warfarin each day
9/08	☐ 2.3	☐ 2.5–3.0	☐ 1.5 mg Warfarin each day
9/11	☐	☐ 2.5–3.0	☐ 2 mg alternating with 1.5 mg Warfarin

Blood pressure refers to the amount of force (pressure) created by the heart as it pumps blood through the arteries. A blood pressure reading consists of two numbers such as 120 over 70 which is read as "120/70." The first or top number (called systolic pressure) is when the heart is working to pump the blood through the arteries. The second or bottom number (called diastolic pressure) is when the heart is at rest and is filling with blood. A person is said to have high blood pressure (HBP) when the top number (systolic) is higher than 140 and/or the bottom number (diastolic) is higher than 85. For persons over age 65, the goal is to maintain pressure no higher than 150/85. Once hypertension is established in older persons, it may not be wise to lower it to 140 since one may need to maintain adequate blood supply to the brain. Your actual goal should be agreed upon with your own physician.

Exercise 6.1 Making a Plan for Myself

1. What is my problem?

- irregular heart beat   _____
- blood clots in my leg   _____
- other   _____

This exercise gives you a chance to score yourself on this item. You can place the date for your "status" at the level where you are now. "Goal" is the level you would like to be at the next time you evaluate yourself along with your nurse or doctor. The next date may be one week or one month or whatever you and your doctor or nurse decide. Early in your treatment after having had a stroke, more frequent checks are done. Later on you may wish to wait longer. At the end of each time you can once again measure your new status and compare it to your goal. You can also see what worked to bring about the change and how much you have contributed to answering these questions.

At first you may just *agree* to the answers your doctor/nurse recommended. Later on you can put *into your own words* what had been recommended. You *confirm your agreement*. Eventually you may be able to *state* for yourself without anyone having to make a recommendation.

2. Following my plan

Participation: Agreement (A) Confirmed Agreement (CA) Statement (S) Specific Statement (SS)			
Date	**Status/Progress**	**Goals**	**What Works**
	☐	☐	☐
	☐	☐	☐

Blood pressure will vary with exercise and stress. When some people go to their doctor, their blood pressure will be higher than usual. The medicine and when you take it will also cause changes in your blood pressure. The only standard condition you can establish is to take your blood pressure at rest and in your home rather than in a doctor's office. The time of day when you take your blood pressure is something to set up with your physician as well as how many times you should take it. It is helpful to bring your blood pressure monitor and your log with you to your doctor's office on occasion to check out its accuracy against one of the standard machines that depend on the use of a stethoscope. You are checking out the machine and also whether you are using it correctly.

When blood pressure becomes too high, a large amount of pressure is put on the walls of the arteries and causes them to weaken. If the pressure continues, this weak spot in the arteries can burst and result in a hemorrhage into the brain. The increased force (pressure) and rate at which the blood is being pushed can also cause hardening and narrowing of the blood vessels over a period of time. Clots can also form that can break loose and plug up an artery and cut off the blood flow to parts of the brain. Hypertension can thus lead to either hemorrhage or blockage. This tends to occur in the small arteries in the brain. Diabetes also tends to increase the likelihood of disease involving these same small vessels.

What Works

What works to reduce blood pressure includes a variety of medicines that cause the blood vessels to widen. As the blood vessels open up, the heart does not have to work as hard to pump the blood, and so the systolic pressure needed also falls. Blood can be pumped throughout the body more easily.

Medicines work in several different ways. The particular medicines recommended by your doctor will vary. Generally, it is helpful to use the fewest different medicines and the fewest total different times to take medicine each day so that it will be easier to remember when to take your medicine and which medicines to take. It is also easier to remember when to refill your medications so that you don't run out. Medicines have effects beyond what may be intended, so that we would like to use as little medication as possible.

Other treatments can help to reduce the need for medicine. You can learn to relax and not let your blood pressure rise. Your blood pressure will rise when you get upset or angry. This is the body's way to get ready to respond to danger. Blood is pumped at a higher rate to the muscles in order to run away or fight. It is called "fight or flight" response. For too many people, this reaction goes on all the time, and the high blood pressure causes all the problems we have described. There may be a need for you to develop other means of dealing with these emotions.

There are other factors to help control blood pressure, such as a diet low in salt. You should avoid canned and pickled foods. It is helpful to check the amount of sodium on labels when food shopping. Weight reduction for overweight patients is also important. Smoking and lack of exercise can cause high blood pressure. Stopping smoking and increasing exercise can help to reduce the chances of a stroke.

When the nurse takes your blood pressure in the hospital, you should ask what are the numbers. You can then decide whether it is too high or not. If it is okay, you can then learn what might be working, including the names of the medication and when and how much you take.

There are blood-pressure machines that give you an automatic reading. These machines enable you to know on your own whether you are meeting your goal. You can learn to use one of them so that you will know how you are doing and can share that information with your physician. Using a cuff around the arm gives you the most accurate reading. Placing a cuff on the forearm can also work. Getting a reading by using your finger is generally not accurate enough, although it is the easiest to do. When you are able to take your own blood pressure at home and know whether it is meeting your goal, you are able to participate with your doctor in reducing the chances of another stroke. It must be stressed how valuable self-monitoring is. When you are reliably measuring your pressure you are taking ownership in your own health.

Making your own plan involves keeping a log of your blood pressure in comparison to the goal and keeping track of your medication as well as your other actions to control blood pressure. It is important to establish with your doctor when you should be concerned about your blood pressure. Then you can then establish when to call to make changes in your medication, diet, or other changes.

Table 6.3 Sample Plan for Managing High Blood Pressure

Date	Status/Progress	Goals	What Actions
9/15	☐ 130/102	☐	☐ HCTZ 25 mg in a.m.; Amlodopine 10 mg in a.m.
9/20	☐ 120/100	☐ Below 140/85	☐ Doxazosin 4 mg p.m.; Amlodopine 10 mg in a.m.
9/23	☐ 120/70	☐ Below 140/85	☐ Doxazosin 5 mg in a.m. and p.m.
9/28	☐	☐ Below 140/85	☐

Table 6.3 describes the log kept by a man with a recent stroke who had high blood pressure. The goal in his case was no higher than 140/85. The two drugs (HCTZ and Autodopine) did not keep his diastolic pressure (the lower number) below 85. Rather than just increasing the doses of the medication he was on, a change was made in the type of medication. The HCTZ was not right for him since it could raise his already high uric acid level and cause him to have an attack of gout. He also had trouble with emptying his urinary bladder. A new drug (Doxazozin) which has a double action was started. It can lower blood pressure and help to empty the bladder. This change in medication eventually worked to control his blood pressure with a single drug, although he was still had to take it twice a day. Sometimes it takes time to find the right drug that works. The type of drug that worked for him was one that not only took care of his high blood pressure but his urinary problems as well.

Exercise 6.2 Making a Plan for Myself

1. What is my problem?

   ● Blood pressure   _____

   Is it less than 140/85 (or 150/85 if more than 65 years old)?
   Exercise 6.2 provides an opportunity to score yourself on this item
   in a way similar to others. You can place the date for your "status"
   alongside the level where you are now. "Goal" is the level you would
   seek to achieve during the interim prior to the next time you evaluate
   yourself along with your nurse or doctor. The next date may be one
   day, one week, or whatever you and your nurse decide. Early in the
   course of your treatment after having had a stroke, frequent intervals
   are used. Later on you may wish to set longer intervals. At the end of
   each interval when you carry out the evaluation along with your nurse,
   you can once again describe your new status and what worked to
   bring about the improvement as well as your goal. Each time you can
   measure your own participation in answering these questions.

   At first you may just *agree* to the answers your doctor/nurse recommend. Later on, you can *put into your own words* what had been recommended. You *confirm your agreement.* Eventually, you may be
   able to *state* for your self without anyone having to make a recommendation.

   2. Following my plan

Participation: Agreement (A) Confirmed Agreement (CA) Statement (S) Specific Statement (SS)			
Date	**Status/Progress**	**Goals**	**What Works**
	☐	☐	☐
	☐	☐	☐

HARDENING OF THE ARTERIES
What is the Problem

One major disease that links many of the risk factors is atherosclerosis or "hardening of the arteries." As a person ages, the arteries harden and fat builds up in the walls of the arteries. This is the cause of disease of the heart and disease of the blood vessels going to the brain. The large arteries that feed the heart and brain are not as elastic, and this loss of "give" in the walls of the arteries makes them "hardened." There can also be ulcers in the fatty build up, and clots can form in these ulcers as well.

There may be blockage by the fatty build up of one of the major blood vessels feeding the brain. Other arteries feeding the brain cannot make up for the blockage since they also have build up and hardening of their walls. Thus, they cannot respond to the blockage that has occurred. These larger arteries can include those that feed the heart muscle. Blockage in the arteries feeding the heart can cause a heart attack because the heart muscle becomes weak and the heart cannot beat regularly. Clots can form in the heart itself and can then go to the brain. There are often similar problems in blood vessels throughout the body. This same blockage can also occur in the blood vessels feeding the legs. Having trouble with your heart or pain in your legs when walking can also be signs of atherosclerosis.

Healthy arteries are flexible like a rubber hose. As fatty build up sticks to the walls, the wall hardens and causes all the arteries to stiffen. Over a period of time, the walls of the smaller arteries also narrow and give the blood less space to flow. To get the blood through the narrow space, the heart must work harder. The amount of force or pressure it takes to push the blood through the arteries is what causes the blood pressure to rise. The smaller arteries in the brain become closed off. This does not allow blood flow to get through to the brain cells and causes a stroke. Hypertension and atherosclerosis combine to increase the damage to the blood vessels.

Too much fat and cholesterol in the diet can increase a person's risk for stroke and heart disease. Dietary cholesterol is found primarily in dairy products and animal fats. Saturated fats are those fats that are solid at room temperature. These fats like butter and many margarines reduce the ability of the body to handle cholesterol effectively and lead to an increased blood level. Atherosclerosis occurs in people that have high levels of fat and cholesterol in the blood (hyperlipidemia). A formation of a soft wax-like substance called plaque builds up along the walls of the arteries.

Each person's liver produces and uses about a gram (or a quarter of a teaspoon) of cholesterol per day. Cholesterol is used in the body to build cells and produce hormones. The combination of fat such as cholesterol and protein is called a lipoprotein. When the blood is tested, certain parts rise to the top because they weigh less or fall to the bottom because they weigh more. For example, low density lipoprotein (LDL) is that portion that rises to the top. About 60%–70% of cholesterol is transported in the form of LDLs and about 20% in the form of high density lipoproteins (HDL) which falls to the bottom.

LDL is called "lousy cholesterol" because it tends to stay in the body and build up in the walls of the arteries. However, not all cholesterol is bad. HDL or high density lipoprotein is called "healthy cholesterol" because it helps to remove the cholesterol that sticks to the arteries. It acts as a vacuum cleaner. The higher your HDL level, the better. Many of the studies you can read about discuss the total cholesterol. A desirable total blood cholesterol level is less than 200 mg (milligrams). Levels between 200 and 239 mg are considered borderline, and 240 mg or above is considered high. In people with stroke or heart disease, it is not enough to measure total cholesterol. It is the parts of your total cholesterol that matter. A lipid profile breaks down that total into its parts. The goals depend on your risk factors. A risk factor is being a man over 45; or a woman over 55. Having a family history of heart disease, being a cigarette smoker, or having high blood pressure or diabetes are also risk factors. The National Institutes of Health (NIH) now recommends that your HDL cholesterol should be above 35 mg/dl and your LDL cholesterol below 100 mg (see Table 6.4). For persons above 70, the guidelines are not as strict.

What Works

What works to reduce LDL is mainly a change in diet. Table 6.5 lists opportunities for changes in your diet that help you to reduce the amount of fat in the blood. If you identify areas where your answer is "often," you can then develop a plan to reduce your use of those categories of foods. A more complete listing of foods is the "Heart

Table 6.4 Range of Lipoprotein Levels

Total	Desirable	Borderline	High
Cholesterol	less than 200 mg/dl	200 - 239 mg/dl	240 mg/dl or above
LDL	less than 100 mg	100 - 130	130 - 160
HDL	more than 35 mg/dl		

Healthy" diet recommended by the American Heart Association in Table 6.6.

There are a number of medications that can help in lowering LDL, if diet alone is not enough. The medications work in different ways. Some work to prevent the fat in the food from getting into the blood. These cause the fat to remain in the stomach and get carried out by the bowels. Others work on the cells in the liver that produce lipids. Some medications work to raise HDL as well as lower LDL. No medication is without side effects, and you want to take only what is neces-

Table 6.5 Opportunities for Dietary Change

How often do you:

	Often	Sometimes	Rarely
1. Drink whole or 2% milk (N/A if don't drink any milk)	____	____	____
2. Eat fried foods?	____	____	____
3. Eat cheeses such as cheddar, American, Swiss? (include cheese containing dishes such as macaroni and cheese and cheeseburgers)	____	____	____
4. Eat sweets such as pastries, donuts, cakes, pies, sweet rolls, chocolate?	____	____	____
5. Eat foods covered in sauces or gravies?	____	____	____
6. Use butter?			
7. Eat hot dogs, bacon, or luncheon meats such as bologna or salami?	____	____	____
8. Eat poultry with the skin on?	____	____	____
9. Eat snacks such as potato chips, taco chips, buttered popcorn, or crackers?	____	____	____

Table 6.6 Diet Changes to Lower Blood Cholesterol Levels

	STEP 1 DIET	
	CHOOSE	**DON'T CHOOSE**
Fish, chicken, turkey, and lean meats	Fish, poultry without skin, lean cuts of beef, lamb, pork, veal, or shellfish	Fatty cuts of beef, lamb, pork; spare ribs; organ meats; regular cold cuts; sausage, hot dogs; bacon; sardines; roe
Skim and low-fat milk, cheese, yogurt, and dairy substitutes	Skim or 1% fat milk (liquid, powdered, evaporated) buttermilk	Whole milk (4% fat); regular, evaporated, condensed; cream; half and half; 2% milk; imitation milk products; most nondairy creamers, whipped toppings
	Nonfat (0% fat) or low-fat yogurt	Whole-milk yogurt
	Low-fat cottage cheese (1% or 2% fat)	Whole-milk cottage cheese (4% fat)
	Low-fat cottage cheeses, farmer or pot cheeses (all of these should be labeled no more than 2 6 g of fat per ounce)	All natural cheeses (e.g., blue Roquefort, Camembert, cheddar, Swiss); low-fat or light" cream cheese; low-fat or "light" sour cream; cream cheeses, sour cream
	Sherbet, sorbet	Ice cream
Eggs	Egg whites (2 whites equal 1 whole egg in recipes), cholesterol-free egg substitutes	Egg yolks
Fruits and vegetables	Fresh, frozen, canned, or dried fruits and vegetables	Vegetables prepared in butter, cream, or other sauces
Breads and cereals	Homemade baked goods using unsaturated oils sparingly, angel food cake, low-fat crackers, low-fat cookies	Commercial baked goods, pies, cakes, doughnuts, croissants, pastries, muffins, biscuits, high-fat crackers, high-fat cookies
	Rice, pasta	Egg noodles
	Whole-grain breads and cereals (oatmeal, wheat, rye, bran, multigrain, etc.)	Breads in which eggs are a major ingredient

Table 6.6 Diet Changes to Lower Blood Cholesterol Levels (Continued)

	STEP 1 DIET	
	CHOOSE	DON'T CHOOSE
Fats and oils	Baking cocoa	Chocolate
	Unsaturated vegetable oils: corn, extra virgin olive, rapeseed (canola oil), safflower, sesame, soybean, sunflower	Butter, coconut oil, palm oil, palm kernel oil, lard, bacon fat
	Margarine or shortening made from one of the unsaturated oils listed previously, low-fat dressings	Dressings made with egg yolk
	Seeds and nuts	Coconut

From National Cholesterol Education Panel: *Arch Int Med* 148:36m 1988.

sary. You should check with your doctor about which medications to use and why.

Exercise is also helpful. People who exercise tend to increase their HDL, the good cholesterol that then helps to reduce the fatty build-up in the arteries. The amount of exercise needed to raise HDL is not entirely clear. Thirty minutes a day of exercise such as walking can make a big difference in your overall health. Making your own plan involves keeping a log of your LDL in comparison to the goal and tracking your medication and/or dietary changes and exercise to control your lipid levels in the blood.

BLOOD SUGAR MANAGEMENT

What is the Problem

The person with diabetes who has had a stroke has two problems. One is the management of the diabetes during the rehabilitation phase. The other is how to prevent another stroke. The problems during the rehabilitation phase are the result of the person with diabetes exercising more than usual. The patient has to work harder when a one has less control of one's limbs. Problems occur when relatively sedentary per-

Exercise 6.3 Making a Plan for Myself

1. What is my problem?

- LDL greater than 100   _____
- HDL less than 35   _____

This exercise gives you a chance to score yourself on this item. You can place the date for your "status" at the level where you are now. "Goal" is the level you would like to be at the next time you evaluate yourself along with your nurse or doctor. The next date may be one week or one month or whatever you and your doctor or nurse decide. Early in your treatment after having had a stroke, more frequent checks are done. Later on you may wish to wait longer. At the end of each time you can once again measure your new status and compare it to your goal. You can also see what worked to bring about the change and how much you have contributed to answering these questions.

At first you may just *agree* to the answers your doctor/nurse recommend. Later on, you can *put into your own words* what had been recommended. You *confirm your agreement*. Eventually, you may be able to *state* for your self without anyone having to make a recommendation.

2. Following my plan

Participation: Agreement (A) Confirmed Agreement (CA) Statement (S) Specific Statement (SS)			
Date	**Status/Progress**	**Goals**	**What Works**
	☐	☐	☐
	☐	☐	☐
	☐	☐	☐

son with a diet and insulin dosage established for rest, suddenly begins exercising. Exercise lowers blood sugar. One goal therefore is to maintain blood sugar in an acceptable range, particularly to prevent too low a blood sugar. The other aspect deals with the effects of diabetes on the person who now exercises. Long-standing diabetes can affect the ability of the nerves in the body to do their work. One set of nerves sends messages back to the brain when the blood sugar is too low. The symptoms vary with the person. Generally, there is sweating, palpitations (rapid heart rate) and a feeling of uneasiness. These symptoms may not, however, be present because the nerves sending these messages may have been damaged. It becomes all the more important to make sure that the blood sugar does not get too low. If your usual goal has been to keep your blood sugar no higher than 100, it might be better to try and keep your average blood sugar no lower than 120.

Another effect of diabetes on the nerves makes it harder for a person to know when the heart is not getting enough blood. There may be insufficient blood going to the heart to keep up with your exercise. The signals one gets again can vary with the person. Some people get a feeling of pressure in the chest or down the arm or get short of breath. These signals of over exertion may not be present due to damage to the nerves that carry the message to the brain. We therefore need to protect against overexertion and act to reduce exertion when any symptoms appear.

Another problem that arises from damage to nerves by diabetes is the control of blood pressure when a person stands up. When you stand up, the heart needs to work harder to get blood to the brain. Because of the damage to the nerves, that response may be delayed and the patient may feel lightheaded. It is necessary to give yourself a longer time to compensate before getting up, particularly after having been in bed for several days or in the morning upon first awakening. These several aspects of the relationship between diabetes and exercise may affect the ability to participate in an active exercise program that is typical in stroke rehabilitation.

Still another goal of managing a person with diabetes and stroke is the prevention of future strokes. The effect of long-standing diabetes is not only on the integrity of the nerves. Even more important is the effect of diabetes on the blood vessels throughout the body. The presence of diabetes typically makes the process of hardening of the arteries even worse. This worsening process occurs even when the blood pressure, cholesterol, and lipid levels are not very high. For persons with microvascular disease, it is particularly important to keep the blood sugar under control. When blood sugar runs high, a chemical is formed that increases even more the tendency for lipids to form on the walls of the arteries. Another important reason to control blood pressure and lipid levels is their impact on the measurements of proteinuria.

Hardening of the arteries is so harmful because it happens throughout the body. It can affect the blood vessels in the eyes and cause blindness, blood vessels in the heart and cause heart attacks, as well as blood vessels in the brain and cause strokes. These problems are less serious when blood sugar is kept as close to normal as possible. The goal, therefore, is to maintain blood sugar within the normal range to prevent the long term complications of diabetes. One way to measure the degree of normality is the percentage of what is called glycosylated hemoglobin. Hemoglobin is the major component of red blood cells. When there is an excess of sugar in the blood, that sugar becomes part of the hemoglobin as it is formed. The goal is to keep that percentage no higher than 7%.

What Works

There are two different kinds of diabetes. The effects on the ability to deal with both the rehabilitation issues and long-term prevention of vascular disease differs with the kind of diabetes you have. Both deal with not enough insulin being available to metabolize sugar in the diet so that it can be stored and work in the cells. Insulin is a chemical produced in the pancreas, an organ near the stomach. Type I diabetes is the term used for persons who generally develop diabetes early in life. They require insulin and can get into trouble when blood sugar is too high. For several different reasons, their pancreas does not produce insulin. Type II diabetes is the more common form and occurs in persons later in life but can also occur in younger people. Type II is more often associated with people who are overweight. There is not enough insulin being produced in the body or the insulin produced is simply not effective. In this instance, some insulin may be produced so that such people are not as dependent on insulin and do not get into as much trouble if the blood sugar is high. Their blood sugar control may need insulin but could also be achieved by oral medicines. In both cases, the treatment includes diet and exercise as well as medicine. It is also important to eat meals and take prescribed medications at the same time every day.

Treatment of Type II diabetes is closely associated with being overweight. Diet control is the most important part of treatment. Many persons find that, with weight under control, the need for medication or insulin becomes much less. The issues to be managed include reducing the total number of calories as well as the distribution of such calories throughout the day. Smaller, more frequent eating can make a difference. The patient must be able to break down the food for energy so that there is not too much food that requires a lot of insulin at once. If there is not too sharp a rise, the body seems be able to keep up with the need. A lower calorie diet can bring the blood sugar under control even before significant weight loss occurs. The total number of calories may vary with the person and the amount of activity or exercise they do. Approximately 12 calories per pound is necessary to maintain weight. If the person weighs 150 pounds, then 1800 calories would be necessary. If the person exercises more actively, then that same weight person would need approximately 2400 calories. Anything less would cause weight loss.

A key aspect of the nutrition is the use of a balanced diet. The amount of protein, fat, and sugars must be adjusted. One can eat some sugar, but more starch than free sugar. The amount of fat should be limited (30%), with reduction in cholesterol and the use of unsaturated fats such as liquid oils. Around 50% of the calories may come from carbohydrates (sugars). Complex carbohydrates are also high in fiber. The information now available on packaged or canned foods can help you select the foods you need for a balanced diet.

The second major aspect of treatment is use of exercise. If the blood sugar is under adequate control, exercise can help to keep it under control with less medication. The recommended amount of exercise is to try to exercise 20 - 30 minutes per day several times a week, with goal of achieving 70% of age adjusted heart rate (220-age). This would help with endurance and heart rate. For example, in a 60-year-old person, the goal would be (220-60) 160 × 70% = 112. Examples of moderate exercise would be walking at 2.5 mph for 30 minutes that would use up 300 calories. Heavy exercise such as cycling (13 mph) would use up 660 calories/hour in a person weighing about 150 pounds.

The third major treatment used when diet and exercise are not enough to control your diabetes is medication. Insulin comes in several forms and the particular dose and form will need to be adjusted to the size of meals and their timing. Each person will need to work this out with his or her doctor. It may be necessary to maintain insulin treatment even in those with Type II diabetes. Insulin requires daily needle injections. There are a number of medications to be taken by mouth that can maintain blood sugar within the normal range in persons with Type II diabetes. The selection of a particular agent should be discussed with your doctor. There are 2 major groups of medication now available.

The sulfonylurea drugs help to release insulin from the pancreas. Glyburide® (Micronase) acts for a longer time than Glipizide® (Glucotrol). Problems can arise from blood sugar falling too low. Since Glipizide® does not last as long, it is less likely to cause a problem. It must generally be given twice a day with meals. Glipizide xl® is longer acting and is given once a day. Metformin® (Glucophage) type drugs act differently. They decrease the amount of sugar made in the liver. They also could cause gastrointestinal upset as a side effect. Acabbose (Precose) is a new drug that slows down the absorption of sugar from the gut after a meal. This allows the pancreas to keep up with the need for insulin. It does not cause the pancreas to produce more insulin, so low blood sugar reactions do not occur. Troglitazone® (Rezulin), Rosiglitazone® (Auand) and Proglitazone® (Actos) are new drugs that makes cells in the body more sensitive to insulin. The major side effect is liver damage, so your physician will check your liver function test.

Judie Gray CRRN, MSN, Adult Nurse Practitioner, collaborated in writing Use of Blood Thinners

Brenda McCall-Russell CRRN collaborated in writing Hypertension Management, Hardening of the Arteries.

Trudy Sellman CRRN collaborated in writing Blood Sugar Management.

Exercise 6.4 Making a Plan for Myself

1. What is the problem

- Blood sugar below 120   _____
- Blood sugar above 180   _____

This exercise gives you a chance to score yourself on this item. You can place the date of your "status" at the level where you are now. "Goal" is the level you would like to be at the next time you evaluate yourself along with your nurse or doctor. The next date may be one day or one week, or whatever your and your doctor or nurse decide. Early during your treatment after having had a stroke, more frequent checks are done. Later on you may wish to wait longer. At the end of each time you can once again measure your new status and compare it to your goal. You can also see what worked to bring about the change and how much you have contributed to answering these questions. We hope that you can answer these questions more and more on your own.

At first you may just *agree* to the answer your doctor/nurse recommend. Later on, you can put into your own words what has been recommended. You *confirm* your *agreement*. Eventually you will be able to *state* for yourself without anyone having to make recommendations.

2. Following my plan

Participation: Agreement (A) Confirmed Agreement (CA) Statement (S) Specific Statement (SS)			
Date	**Status/Progress**	**Goals**	**What Works**
	☐	☐	☐
	☐	☐	☐
	☐	☐	☐

—7—

Communication and Swallowing Problems

CHRISTINE BARON

When there are communication
and swallowing problems after stroke, the effects can be devastating.
Eating contributes to our sense of well being and is often part of social
gatherings. Communication skills help us maintain our sense of
ourselves. We use communication to learn, gain support, and—in general—to adjust to change. Problems with communication and swallowing can make the process of adjusting to change after stroke more
difficult. Evaluation and treatment of communication and swallowing
problems by a speech-language pathologist (SLP) can maximize recovery of these important skills and improve the whole rehabilitation
process. The end of this chapter (Table 7.1) contains a log for the patient with stroke to write down the goals, problems, questions, and successes that are experienced when striking back at stroke.

COMMUNICATION PROBLEMS

Changes in communication abilities after stroke are common. These
changes can cause mild, moderate, or severe problems. The degree to
which stroke-related communication changes will affect a person's
functioning depends in part on how much the person used communication skills in everyday life before he or she had a stroke. Even mild
communication changes can sometimes have a significant effect on a
person's ability to go back to activities enjoyed before the stroke. At
the same time, moderate communication changes don't necessarily
keep a person from resuming many pre-stroke activities, with help
from a speech-language pathologist. Stroke can affect communication
in many ways. It is common for a person to have more than one kind
of communication problem after a stroke.

Aphasia

The word system used to communicate is called language. Speakers of Spanish language, for instance, use different words to communicate from the words used by speakers of English. The words spoken or written in Spanish are different from those in English because it's a different language. Language matches meaning with words so people can communicate.

Aphasia is a loss of language skill that can happen after a stroke. Language skills include speaking, understanding what is heard (or auditory comprehension), reading, and writing. Aphasia impairs all of these to some degree. Usually, the amount of impairment in each of these areas is different. For example, some people with aphasia have more trouble talking than understanding what is said to them. Other people with aphasia speak easily, but they don't understand very well what they hear.

For most people, aphasia comes from a stroke on the left side of the brain. That's because most people are right-handed, and most right-handed people have language skills located on the left side of the brain. People who are left-handed can have aphasia from a stroke on the right side of the brain. The kind of stroke that causes aphasia most often makes the dominant (usually right) hand and arm weak or paralyzed.

The language skills that are the most impaired by aphasia depend on which part of the brain had the stroke. Strokes in the front of the brain tend to impair talking more than auditory comprehension. Strokes in the back of the brain tend to impair auditory comprehension more than talking. Most people with aphasia have more trouble with reading and writing than they do with talking and understanding. When someone has aphasia, he has trouble doing things involving words. For example, the person with aphasia has a harder time remembering something he is told how to do than something he is shown how to do. Because aphasia is a problem with words, any activity that uses words may be harder than before the stroke.

Some people with aphasia have a lot of trouble understanding what others say to them. Some people with aphasia understand things that are said to them quite well. When a person with aphasia has good comprehension, families often think that they understand everything. This is very rarely the case. When there is noise (a television or radio), a conversation of several speakers or the topic of conversation changes fast, most people with aphasia will have some trouble understanding. Full comprehension may also be difficult if the person with aphasia is tired.

People with aphasia have trouble putting their thoughts into words. The problem in aphasia isn't thinking of what to say, but saying it. Some people with aphasia speak easily, but don't always make a lot of sense. Some people with aphasia have trouble getting any words to come out at all. They may say a word that is closely related in meaning to the one they want to say. For example, "blue" can be easily said instead of "green," or "sister" said instead of "daughter." Words that sound alike, such as "pork" for "fork" might also be substituted for each other by a person with aphasia.

People with aphasia communicate better if they are in the situation or context that is being talked about. People with aphasia can see and use many visual cues in a context to help express themselves or understand what is said. Information in the form of gestures or pictures is easier than words for people with aphasia to understand. Sometimes, people with aphasia can draw and use gestures or pictures to communicate quite well.

Cognitive-Communication Disorder

Cognitive-communication skills are the way we use thinking to communicate. To communicate well, we need to be able to see and concentrate on what is going on around us. We need to remember things and think things through, sometimes quite fast. For example, when deciding if people should be introduced, we need to remember if we have ever introduced them or it's likely they've met before. Often this kind of quick thinking goes on without our awareness. We adjust our tone of voice, facial expression, and when/how often we speak to coordinate with the person talked to. The way we talk to a person depends on if we've talked to them before and how well we know them. We use humor with some people (especially family and friends), but choose not to with others. We communicate a lot with our tone of voice and body language.

Cognitive-communication disorder after a stroke is the loss of the ability to see and concentrate on what is happening around us during communication. Changes with memory and the ability to put things together to make decisions are part of this problem. The exact pattern of problems is different for each person with cognitive-communication disorder. Because basic communication is often not impaired, people with cognitive-communication disorder may not realize that they have communication problems in more complicated situations.

Cognitive-communication disorder can come from a stroke on either side of the brain, but most of the time, it comes from a stroke on the right side of the brain. That's because most people are right-handed and most right-handed people have attention, concentration, memory, and putting things together controlled by the right side of the brain. People who are left handed can have cognitive-communication disorder from a stroke on the left side of the brain. The kind of stroke that causes cognitive-communication disorder most often makes the non-dominant (usually left) hand and arm weak, if the body has weakness from the stroke.

People with a cognitive-communication disorder usually have trouble concentrating on and making sense of what they see. Often, people with cognitive-communication disorder don't pay attention to things that are on one side. This is called neglect and is frequently neglect of things on the left. When a person with neglect reads, one side of the page may not totally be seen. Sometimes, it's the one side of individual words that are read wrong or not seen. The problem is not with vision, but with attention. Besides not concentrating on what they're seeing on one side, people with neglect also may not respond to what they hear or feel on the neglected side. It's as though their full awareness doesn't go all the way over to the neglected side anymore. Concentrating on things on the neglected side seems to be as hard for people with neglect as it would be for anyone to concentrate on what is happening over their shoulder. It would take us extra energy and effort always to concentrate on what is happening over the shoulder. So also, it takes a lot of energy and effort for people with neglect to pay attention to things in their neglected area.

Cognitive-communication disorder often makes it harder for a person to concentrate on what he hears especially if he needs to listen for a long time. The person with cognitive-communication disorder may start listening to a story or explanation and lose focus part way through. This can lead to misunderstanding or poor memory. People with cognitive-communication disorder can also misunderstand things that others don't come right out and say. We often expect others to figure out what we mean by our tone of voice, body language, or the situation. For example, if we say "I'm tired" early in the morning, we may expect to be offered a cup of coffee. If we say the same thing late at night, we may expect to be left alone to relax or to go to bed. People with cognitive-communication disorder can have trouble figuring things out when they are communicating. They do better if people say just what they mean. The same changes in attention and thinking that cause problems for listening comprehension can cause problems for reading comprehension, too.

Cognitive-communication disorder makes it hard for a person to communicate well. He may talk without awareness of the listener by talking too quickly to be understood or by saying things said before. Sometimes the tone of voice and face lack expression (the person looks flat). Some people with cognitive-communication disorder talk non-stop. Some people with cognitive-communication disorder don't say much at all unless questioned. People with cognitive-communication may come across in ways they don't intend. Because they have trouble taking in everything going on around them and making good decisions with the information while they're communicating. Sometimes, people with cognitive-communication disorder make quick decisions (impulsivity) without taking everything into consideration. Sometimes, people with cognitive-communication disorder don't initiate asking for something that they need.

People who have a cognitive-communication disorder don't usually have much trouble communicating basic things, but they may have trouble communicating more complicated things. They are also good at picking out the details, but they may have trouble pulling everything together into a whole in order to solve a problem or make a decision.

Dysarthria

Speech is the way we sound when we talk. When a person has a cold, speech sounds different because a stuffy nose won't let sound go through or a sore throat makes the voice sound different. Speech involves breathing, making sound in the voice box, sending that sound through the mouth or nose, and moving the tongue and lips to create words. All of these things happen because the different groups of muscles that control these skills move together to make speech.

Dysarthria is a change in the sound or clearness of speech that can happen after a stroke. Speech can sound different because of changes in the way the muscles of the mouth, throat, and face move. Muscles can lose strength or the ability to move fully or smoothly. Sometimes, the problem is the coordination between the muscles. The melody of the speech can be changed. Often, speech is slurred, and it needs to be repeated to be understood. In severe cases, no sound can be made at all, or sometimes sounds are so far off that they can't be understood, even with repetition.

Dysarthria comes from a stroke on either side of the brain or from a stroke to the back part of the brain called the brainstem. The kind of stroke that causes dysarthria can make muscles weak, tight, or unable to move smoothly on either side of the body. When someone has dysarthria, there is often involvement of body muscles. When a person has dysarthria after a stroke, he also often has trouble swallowing (dysphagia). Some of the same muscles that control speech also control swallowing.

When someone has dysarthria, it is difficult to speak the same way as before the stroke. The person with dysarthria may speak too softly or loudly. The voice may sound gravely, breathy, or higher or lower pitched than before. Often, speakers with dysarthria have trouble being understood by other people. They know what they want to say, but just have trouble being understood.

Some dysarthric speakers can repeat or make small changes to the way they speak, so that they are understood. Because the average person doesn't think that much about the way they sound when speaking, learning to talk differently can take a lot of practice and therapy.

When dysarthria is more severe, sometimes people need another way to communicate to use along with their speech or instead of their speech. Writing, gestures, pictures, a letter board, or an electronic "talker" can be used by a speaker with dysarthria when speech alone doesn't work completely.

Speakers with dysarthria communicate best if they look right at the listener when they talk. Sometimes the listener will understand part, but not all of what was said. If the listener says the part that was understood, that technique will help the speaker with dysarthria repeat only the part that wasn't understood. Speaking can take a lot of effort for some speakers with dysarthria. Letting them know which part of the message you didn't understand will help them conserve energy and communicate to the best of their ability.

Apraxia of Speech

The muscles that produce speech need to move together in a pattern or sequence in order to form sounds or words. This movement happens very quickly, without much thought.

The movement happens over and over again, without failure. The brain sends messages to the muscles of speech and tells them to move in certain patterns to make sounds and words, such as to close the lips to make a "p" sound or the word "pepper."

Apraxia of speech is a loss of the ability to make sequenced patterns of movements for talking. This can happen after stroke. When someone is apraxic, the message sent from the brain is changed by the time it reaches the muscles. For example, the brain may have thought of and sent the word "tornado" to the muscles used for speech. Apraxia of speech might cause the word to be spoken "tordeeno" or "taydorno." In each case, the message sent by the brain gets jumbled by the time it reaches the speech muscles.

For most people, apraxia of speech comes from a stroke on the left side of the brain. That's because most people are right-handed and most right-handed people have muscle movement patterns for speech located on the left side of the brain. People who are left-handed can have apraxia of speech from a stroke on the right side of the brain. When someone has apraxia of speech, there is often involvement of body muscles. The kind of stroke that causes apraxia of speech most often makes the dominant (usually right) hand and arm weak or apraxic.

Apraxia of speech is like a glitch in the speech system. Sometimes the correct sounds or words will be spoken without difficulty, and the next time, they are jumbled or wrong. The problem is in the sending of the message from the brain to the muscles. The problem isn't in thinking of what to say or with the muscles themselves. It is common for a person with apraxia to say something well, and then not be able to repeat what he just said. Usually, people with apraxia show a lot of struggle and effort when talking. When apraxia of speech is severe, it is hard for people to say anything at all, much like the person with severe dysarthria.

When someone has apraxia of speech, he has more trouble saying something if he is concentrating on his speech. The more a person with apraxia tries to speak correctly, the harder it is to speak. Sometimes, he repeats things, but a different wrong word comes out each time. Simple sequences of words that we learned long ago, such as counting or the days of the week, often are spoken most easily. Common phrases such as "I'm fine" or "I don't know" may also come more easily. However, a sentence as basic as "My name is Bob" can be very difficult for a person with apraxia to say, because it is not automatic. The person with apraxia knows what he wants to say, he just has trouble saying it.

When apraxia is more severe, people may need another way to communicate that they use with their speech or instead of their speech. Writing, gestures, pictures, a letter board or an electronic "talker" can be used by people with apraxia when they cannot communicate with speech alone.

Speakers with apraxia talk best when they don't think too much about talking. When they have trouble saying something, their listeners or they may want to take the focus off of talking. That approach can be helpful. Sometimes, the word pops out when another form of communication (writing, pictures) is used.

EVALUATION OF COMMUNICATION DISORDERS

Because strokes affect communication abilities differently for each person, an evaluation of communication after stroke needs to be different for each person. No two evaluations are exactly the same, just as no two people have exactly the same kind of communication problems after stroke. The SLP will figure out which tests to use and how long the testing needs to go on. Most evaluations are a combination of formal and informal tests. Usually, a thorough evaluation takes about three one-hour sessions

Evaluation of communication abilities after stroke is done for many reasons. The SLP needs to determine the presence or absence of aphasia, cognitive-communication disorder, dysarthria, and/or apraxia. Family members or friends can be especially helpful during the evaluation process by helping the SLP understand how the stroke survivor was communicating and what he enjoyed doing before the stroke. It's important for the SLP to know which problems are new, and if any problems were there before the stroke (such as a hearing or memory problem)

When communication problems are found, the severity of each one is determined as part of the evaluation. A communication evaluation will determine the prognosis or likelihood of recovery of communication function. Because communication strengths and weaknesses are discovered during the evaluation, it will also be the starting point for treatment. During the evaluation, many different therapy techniques are tried to see how the stroke survivor responds.

TREATMENT OF COMMUNICATION DISORDERS

Treatment of communication problems after a stroke is done by a certified SLP. An SLP Assistant can provide treatment when working under the supervision of a certified SLP. Families, friends, and volunteers can also be an important part of the therapy plan that the SLP develops. Treatment should start as soon as possible after a stroke. What is done during treatment depends on what was discovered during the evaluation. Like the evaluation, each person's treatment plan is different and is designed just for him. Families and friends should learn the specific treatment techniques from the SLP. Therapy plans are updated every week in the beginning, and every month later on. Therapy includes both stimulation and compensation techniques.

Stimulation refers to the "exercising" of a certain skill to make it better or stronger. For example, doing a drill where someone helps a stroke survivor say a list of words or answer a list of questions is stimulation therapy. Like doing sit-ups, the more the drill is practiced, the better the result will be. The amount of time that a person spends with an SLP each day is at most an hour. For stimulation therapy to work best, families, friends, or stroke survivors themselves need to do the practice drill outside of the SLP treatment sessions.

Compensation refers to finding a way to work around a lost skill. For example, when someone can't say what he wants to say, he can learn to use a communication board of pictures or words. In this way, he compensates for the trouble he has talking, and succeed in communicating. While SLPs work on compensation techniques in treatment, families and friends can help here too. By learning what compensation techniques a stroke survivor is using, families and friends can encourage the use of these techniques whenever the stroke survivor is communicating. Often families are active participants in the individual therapy with the SLP and the stroke survivor. The use of compensation techniques takes practice. The more places and people the stroke survivor can practice with, the better.

Group therapy should be included as part of the communication treatment plan as soon as possible. One of the special benefits of group therapy is the greater number of communication partners. The greater the number of people with whom a stroke survivor practices communication techniques, the better the use of those techniques will be. Besides a chance to practice the therapy techniques, the stroke survivor can learn what works for others.

Communication recovery continues over many months and years. The amount of change in each past week/month is a good predictor of the amount of recovery to expect in the next week/month. Recovery is greater in the beginning, and slows down with time. In the beginning, stroke survivors can have as much as one hour of communication therapy a day. As communication recovery slows down, and as the stroke survivor is able to do the therapy techniques outside of the SLP treatment session (often with family or friends), formal treatment with an SLP occurs less often.

Often today, payment for communication therapy is terminated by the insurer before the stroke survivor has reached the maximum benefit from SLP treatment. When this happens, the stroke survivor may continue to pay out-of-pocket for SLP treatment. Group treatment is sometimes provided at a lower cost, and may be more affordable when insurance payments stop before therapy is completed. Finally, getting treatment from an SLP graduate training program at an area university may be a lower-cost option for continued SLP treatment.

No matter where a stroke survivor is in communication recovery, he should consider joining a stroke club. The supportive atmosphere

---

**Suggestions for Helping Someone Who Has
Communication Problems Following a Stroke**

- Be patient. It often takes longer to communicate after stroke.
- Communicate face to face. The listener can pick up clues other than the words (mouth shape, facial expression).
- Look for other ways to communicate if using words doesn't work (pictures, gestures, facial expression, tone of voice).
- Relax and listen. Often what is spoken is close to the actual message. If you relax, you'll be better at figuring out what was said.
- Don't be afraid or embarrassed to say you didn't understand. Don't pretend to understand if you don't. Ask questions or ask for clarification if you're not sure what was communicated.
- If communication has failed and frustration is high, ask if you can "let it go for now."
- Make the environment as quiet and distraction free as possible. Turn off the T.V. Ask children to play in another room.
- Have your hearing evaluated or get a hearing aid, if you have been putting it off or think you might benefit from one. You may be missing sounds that would let you figure out some messages.
- If you're not sure that you were understood, repeat or give the stroke survivor a chance to show you that he understood.
- Don't talk as though the stroke survivor can't understand. Even when there is a severe problem with comprehension, the stroke survivor may understand some of what you're saying.
- Watch out for overloading the stroke survivor. When he looks tired, help him find a way to take a break or a nap.
- Don't ask a stroke survivor to do two things at the same time.
- Talk to the speech-language pathologist working with your family member or friend to find out exactly how you can help with communication and recovery.
- Consider using the log sheet at the end of this chapter to record your goals, questions, problems, and successes.

---

of a stroke club is an ideal place both to practice communicating and to continue to learn about stroke and meet other people.

SWALLOWING PROBLEMS

Changes in swallowing abilities after stroke are common, especially in the first few days after stroke. These changes can cause problems so severe that a feeding tube is needed to maintain healthly intake of food and liquid. Less severe changes may require the stroke survivor to eat a special diet or eat in a different way. While swallowing recovers, finding the best way for a stroke survivor to safely eat and drink is the aim of evaluation and treatment. Most people who have dysphagia after stroke recover at least some ability to eat and drink safely.

Dysphagia

Eating involves using mouth and throat muscles to chew and swallow food or to drink liquid. Without thinking much about it, we move the food or liquid through our mouths, close off our windpipe, and swallow it completely. Sometimes food or liquid "goes down the wrong pipe" or goes into the airway, and we cough or choke. Most of the time though, the many muscles work together in a sequenced, coordinated way for smooth chewing and swallowing.

Dysphagia is the loss of ability to chew and/or swallow safely and smoothly and can happen after a stroke. Dysphagia happens because of changes in the way the muscles of the mouth and throat work. Muscles can lose strength or the ability to move fully or smoothly. Sometimes, the problem is the coordination between different muscle movements. Often, swallowing is not safe unless special techniques are used when eating or drinking. In severe cases, feeding tubes in the stomach or nose are used when swallowing cannot be done well enough or safely enough by mouth.

Dysphagia comes from a stroke on either side of the brain or from a stroke to the back part of the brain called the brainstem. The kind of stroke that causes dysphagia can make muscles weak, tight, or unable to move smoothly on either side of the body. When someone has dysphagia, there is often involvement of body muscles. When a person has dysphagia after a stroke, he often also has dysarthria (trouble with speech). Some of the same muscles that control speech also control swallowing.

When someone has dysphagia, he has trouble eating and drinking the same way he did before their stroke. Problems can happen in the mouth with chewing, keeping food in the mouth, or clearing the mouth. Sometimes, the tongue has trouble getting the food or liquid in position to swallow. Often, throat muscles are weak or incoordinated, and food or liquid goes into the airway or remains in the throat after the swallow. Sometimes the voice sounds wet.

People with dysphagia may need to eat special diets and/or use techniques to make their swallow work better. When recommended techniques are not used, people with swallowing problems may be taking the risk of getting food and liquid in the airway and getting a lung infection (pneumonia). Coughing is a reflex that happens when food or liquid goes into the airway. If the cough is weak, pneumonia may develop more easily. Some people with dysphagia don't cough at all when food or liquid goes into their airway. This is called silent aspiration, and can be very dangerous. When dysphagia is more severe, feeding tubes may be needed. Tube feedings can be helpful when the stroke survivor has silent aspiration or is unable to eat and drink enough to stay healthy. Usually, feeding tubes (nose or stomach) are temporary and help to keep the stroke survivor healthy while swallowing recovers.

People with dysphagia do best when they are not rushed through meals. Eating and drinking often take longer with dysphagia. Giving a little extra time can make all the difference between success and failure. Patience is important for the both family and the stroke survivor.

Evaluation of Dysphagia

An evaluation of swallowing disorders after stroke is usually done by an SLP. SLPs are trained to know how the muscles of the mouth and throat work. Many of the same muscles used for speaking are also used for swallowing. In some health care settings, occupational therapists evaluate swallowing in addition to feeding.

Because strokes affect swallowing in a different way for each person, an evaluation of swallowing after stroke needs to be different for each person. Evaluation can be done while watching the stroke survivor eat snacks or a meal. A swallowing study can also be done in radiology. This is indicated when there is a question of how well the throat is working. This test is called a modified barium swallowing study and is like an x-ray video. This is the most common way to find out if there is silent aspiration. The SLP and the radiologist can actually see the stroke survivor swallow and determine if there is a problem.

A swallowing evaluation is done to figure out if there are chewing and swallowing problems in the mouth and throat. Problems in the mouth are called oral dysphagia. Problems in the throat are called pharyngeal dysphagia (pharynx is the medical term for the throat). Family members and friends can be especially helpful during the evaluation process by helping the SLP understand how the stroke survivor chewed and swallowed before the stroke. It's important for the SLP to know which problems are new, and if any problems were there before the stroke.

When swallowing problems are found, the severity is determined as part of the evaluation. A swallowing evaluation will determine the prognosis or likelihood of recovery of swallowing function. A swallowing evaluation is the starting point for swallowing treatment. During the evaluation, many different therapy techniques are tried to see how the stroke survivor responds.

Treatment of Dysphagia

Treatment of dysphagia after a stroke is done by a certified SLP. An SLP Assistant can provide treatment when working under the supervision of a certified SLP. Families, friends, and volunteers can also be an important part of the therapy plan that the SLP develops. Treatment should start as soon as possible after a stroke. What is done during treatment depends on what was discovered during the evaluation. Each person's treatment plan is different and is designed just for him. Families and friends should learn the specific treatment techniques from the SLP. Therapy plans are updated every week in the beginning, and every month later on. Therapy is made up of both stimulation and compensation techniques.

Stimulation refers to the "exercising" of a certain skill to make it better or stronger. For example, doing exercises to make the tongue or lips work better is stimulation therapy. Like doing sit-ups, the more the exercise is practiced, the better the result will be. The amount of time that a person spends with an SLP each day, is at most, an hour. For stimulation therapy to work the best, families, friends, or the stroke survivor themselves need to practice the exercises outside of the SLP treatment sessions. A common kind of stimulation therapy for the muscles of swallowing is just the act of swallowing itself. Often techniques are needed in order for the swallowing to be done safely.

Compensation refers to finding a way to work around a lost skill. For example, when someone tucks their head when they swallow, he is compensating for not being able to swallow well without this tech-

> ### Suggestions for Helping Someone Who Has Dysphagia Following a Stroke
>
> - Allow extra time for eating and drinking.
> - Be sure the person with dysphagia is seated upright in a chair when he is eating or drinking.
> - Take care that the person with dysphagia doesn't lie down for about thirty minutes after a meal.
> - Don't carry on a conversation with the person with dysphagia while he is eating or drinking.
> - Talk to the SLP working with your family member or friend to find out exactly how you can help with swallowing and recovery.
> - Consider using the log sheet at the end of this chapter to record your goals, questions, problems and successes.

nique. In this way, he compensates for the trouble in swallowing, and succeeds at eating or drinking. While SLPs work on compensation techniques in treatment, families and friends can help. By learning what compensation techniques a stroke survivor is using, families and friends can encourage the use of these techniques whenever the stroke survivor is eating or drinking. The use of compensation techniques takes practice. The more the stroke survivor practices, the better.

A common compensation for dysphagia is changing the kinds of food or liquid that a person eats and drinks. In general, the thicker something is (applesauce is thicker than water), the easier it is for a person with dysphagia to swallow it. That is because thicker things move more slowly in the throat and are less likely to get into the airway. Thickening liquid, sometimes so it is as thick as pudding, is common after stroke. The body uses this thickened liquid to stay healthy in the same way it uses normal liquid. Sometimes, chewing is a problem. Putting food in the blender or chopping it can make it easier for the mouth to handle the food.

People with dysphagia do best when they use their techniques or diet modifications when they are eating and drinking. Family members and friends can help by encouraging the use of the techniques and not giving the stroke survivor food or liquid that is not safe. As swallowing recovers, techniques may not be needed. It's important to use the techniques needed until recovery makes them unnecessary.

Table 7.1 Making a Plan for Myself

1. What are my problems?

The answers to the question and the problems are yours to describe. The problem you may have depends on your own particular situation and your concerns.

1. _____
2. _____
3. _____

The answers to the question of goals are also yours to describe. It is helpful not only to specify what you wish to accomplish, but how much, or how fast, or how independently. When answering the question about what results you find have been achieved, it is helpful to specify not only what the results were but where or when it happened. The answers to the question about what works may also be your ideas or equipment you have found useful. It is helpful not only to specify what you do to contribute to the results, but how you go about it. "How often" or "where" or "when" are some additional questions to help make your statements more specific.

2. Following my plan

Participation: Agreement (A) Confirmed Agreement (CA) Statement (S) Specific Statement (SS)			
Date	Status/Progress	Goals	What Works
	☐	☐	☐
	☐	☐	☐
	☐	☐	☐
	☐	☐	☐

—8—

Physical Recovery, Daily Living Skills, And Equipment Issues Across the Continuum of Care

MARTHA CARROLL
GRETCHEN BRAUN VIDERGAR

Recovery from a stroke is difficult to explain or predict since each person may have different problems and different weaknesses. In addition to the many problems one experiences following a stroke, there are many strengths that have not been lost. Enlist family and friends in assisting to build up those strengths and to reinforce progress daily. Keep in mind that it took many years to develop the strengths that have now been lost; rebuilding them will take time as well. This chapter will begin with an outline of the problems related to stroke recovery and is followed by the effects these problems have on activities of daily living and functional mobility. We also discuss equipment interventions and some common stroke recovery strategies. At the end of this chapter Table 8.1 contains a log for the patient to write down the goals, problems, questions, and successes that are experienced when striking back at stroke.

PHYSICAL CHANGES/IMPAIRMENTS

Vision

There are many changes that may occur with visual and perceptual processes as a result of stroke. Some of these changes have to do with the actual visual system, and others have to do with the visual processing systems in the brain. Due to an interruption of the visual pathways in the brain, there may be loss of parts or all of what are called visual

153

fields. Loss of half of a field in one eye is called a hemianopsia; loss of half the fields in both eyes is called homonymous hemianopsia. A person will often say that things come up quickly on one side, or that he bumps into things on one side when experiencing these problems. These losses in vision can be compensated for easily by re-learning how to look for things in the environment so that the missing visual field is always checked for obstacles. For example, a person missing the left lower field of vision may start to look for things in a room or in a drawer by always starting in the lower left corner. By changing the way in which a person gets visual information, this problem can essentially disappear.

Visual Perception

Neglect is often discussed in relation to a visual field loss and is a loss of awareness of body parts or objects on one side of the body. It is usually seen when weakness is on the left side. Neglect may be present even when the visual field is not impaired. Neglect can be quite challenging for not only the individual experiencing it, but his or her family members as well. The information the brain receives does not include information about the left side, so the person neglects that side. A person who has neglect will often need someone to ask him to turn his head to look to the affected side. During meals, he may eat food on only one side of his plate and not notice dessert in the upper left corner of his tray. He may not make eye contact with a visitor who has just come into the room from the left, but he will carry on a conversation.

There are many ways to help someone with neglect. One is to sit toward the side the person neglects to encourage head turning and making eye contact. During meals, instruct the person to trace the outside of his plate, or name all of the objects on his tray so that he knows what is there to eat. One can also cue the patient to turn his head to look for things, but remember to make sure his eyes are moving also. Lastly, one can keep a red line on the table, or on the object he is working with to give the person recovering from stroke a target from where to start looking for things around him.

Another common perceptual problem is determining relationships of objects to each other or distinguishing parts of objects as part of the whole object. A person who cannot tell a shirtsleeve from the body of the shirt will have trouble putting it on. A person who cannot determine the relationship of the cap to the toothpaste tube will have trouble putting the top back on. Someone who has difficulty determining the right from the left, or the top from the bottom, will have difficulty finding things in a closet or on a shelf. These can present problems when it comes to feeding, and dressing; they can get in the way of being able to safely drive and manage a wheelchair in a new or cluttered environment.

Perceptual Motor

Another common problem seen in stroke rehabilitation is apraxia. There are a variety of different types, but generally this is a problem with performing purposeful movements; it is commonly seen in grooming and feeding tasks, and may occur in transfers. The person who has had a stroke may pick up a toothbrush, wanting to brush his teeth, and proceed to take the toothbrush to his hair and start brushing. Sometimes, he may know that what he has done is not the correct movement for the toothbrush, but he cannot coordinate to do the movement correctly. Other times he may not know how the toothbrush should be used. Apraxia is difficult to explain, and can be very hard for both the one who has had the stroke and his caregiver. Typically, guiding movements can help to reestablish old patterns, and practice in a real situation can assist individuals with apraxia to relearn how to do their daily living tasks again.

Cognition

There are many cognitive changes that can occur with stroke. Two of the more readily noticed are problems with attention and memory. Problems with attention interfere with being able to stay on topic in a conversation, to learn new information, and to complete started tasks. Problems with memory are noticed in poor recall for daily events, new techniques, and new information in general. However, individuals can generally recall long-term information following a stroke, such as addresses, phone numbers, and important people.

There are other cognitive changes often seen following stroke. Problem-solving abilities may be limited, so developing new ways to do things or to do old things differently may require some assistance. Initiating things that once came naturally, such as eating at mealtime, or getting ready in the morning may need some extra prompting following a stroke. One other problem often seen is self monitoring, or taking notice of one's self, one's performance, and one's surroundings. Problems here can affect one's ability to safely do the normal activities, from feeding to dressing. The patient may not be checking his position or his safety along the way.

Sensation

The physical problems related to stroke recovery often interfere with daily tasks, or can at least make them more difficult. One of these problems is difficulty with sensation; this can be sensation contact with objects or knowing where one's body parts are in space. After a stroke, sensory information may not be reliably transmitted to the brain. This may put the person who has had a stroke in danger in some situations.

Everyone relies on input from their environment to assist him or her in making adjustments to normal activities. Feeling a warm burner prompts one to use an oven mitt. Being able to sense contact with objects is essential to being able to walk safely and work in a kitchen without being burned. Although someone with impaired sensation may still be able to move the affected arm and leg, the movement may not be automatic or it may be uncoordinated. The patient may not be able to feel the position of the arm or leg as the person with stroke puts on his shirt or pants. He may also have difficulty knowing where to place his foot as he walks. As the body recovers from the stroke, some or all of the lost sensation may return. In the meantime, therapists can provide strategies that can help someone with a loss of sensation manage to complete daily living and mobility tasks. One suggestion is to use his or her vision. Looking at the position of the arm or leg during an activity is often a very effective way of working with a sensory loss.

Motor Control

One of the most obvious ways someone is affected by a stroke is in the ability to move. The amount of movement, the quality and strength of the movement someone has after a stroke depends upon what part of the brain has been affected and whether the stroke was due to a blockage or a bleed. Some people are able to move both arm and leg, while others can move either the arm or leg, but not both.

Another part of the body that is usually affected is the trunk. The trunk is the mid-section of the body and stretches from chest to pelvic area. A strong or stable trunk makes it easier for the patient to move the arms and legs. A weak trunk makes it more difficult for someone who has suffered a stroke to move his arms and legs, especially on the weak side. It also makes balancing in standing or sitting more difficult as well.

Motor control relates to one's ability to adjust one's body while reaching for things on the floor or reaching to put something on a shelf. After a stroke, when muscles are weak, other muscles will over-power the weak ones because the person is trying so hard to perform a movement. Without a balance of power, controlled movement is difficult to perform so muscle groups may work together to control movement. This results in movements not typical to what seems normal movement. With the help of therapy, the trunk as well as the affected arm and leg can be strengthened and normal movement patterns can be performed. This will allow the person who has suffered a stroke to more easily complete daily living and functional mobility tasks.

Balance/Coordination

Because of the imbalance in muscle strength between the stronger and weaker side of the body, persons who have suffered strokes often have difficulty maintaining their balance in sitting and/or standing. Activities like sitting at the edge of the bed, coming to standing, moving from one surface to another, and walking may be very difficult. Problems with balance may be complicated by problems of decreased sensation, perception, or vision. It may also be difficult for the person who has suffered a stroke to coordinate movement of his arm and leg. This loss makes use of the limbs uncontrolled and inefficient for functional mobility and activities of daily living.

Attaining balance in both a sitting and standing position is critical to being able to complete tasks both safely and efficiently. As the trunk and the weaker arm and leg become stronger and as one's ability to know when he is sitting or standing upright returns, mobility tasks become easier.

DAILY LIVING SKILLS

The primary objective of occupational therapy with persons who have had a stroke is to return them to their normal daily lives and routines. Therapists strive to assist individuals in returning to these routines without special adaptations or equipment, but when it is possible to provide a piece of equipment to facilitate someone's independence, that is the next best choice.

Feeding

Safe feeding is often a major concern for someone who has had a stroke. One side of the muscles used for swallowing may be paralyzed. Then the person is at risk for food travelling down the airway into the lungs and causing pneumonia. Safe feeding depends on good motor control and postural control, good sensation to feel food on the outside of one's mouth, good coordination and the ability to properly use utensils, the ability to see the food on the plate, and good self awareness. Therapists may use techniques such as guiding with their hands to help ease movement from plate to mouth; they may also give the person strategies to put their fork down between each bite to slow them down to enable a safe swallow. Therapists may also ask patients what food is in front of them to make sure they are aware of all areas of the plate or tray. Often a therapist will remind the patient to start looking on one side of the tray where he may consistently forget to find things. Persons recovering from a stroke may not have sensation on one side of the face and may need reminders to wipe that side of the face every one or two bites. These strategies are easily carried over at home and can be reinforced by family or friends.

Some equipment often provided for those experiencing weakness on one side and unable to cut is a rocker knife. This kind of knife is designed for one-handed cutting and assists the patient with independently cutting food. At times, a plate guard or a rimmed plate may be provided to assist with scooping food up off of the plate with one hand. Although there are a wide variety of adaptations possible, these are two of the more common ones.

Grooming

Many of the same problems that interfere with feeding play a part in the difficulties experienced with grooming. One needs good strength, visual skills, perceptual skills, motor planning, and motor control to safely perform grooming tasks such as applying deodorant, make-up, shaving, brushing teeth, and combing and styling one's hair. Again, some of the strategies are the same as those used in feeding: guiding one's hand to his hair or his teeth and then letting the patient take over. The patient can use a mirror as a final check on the outcome and can use one-handed techniques to open containers and apply make-up, toothpaste, and deodorant.

There are a few pieces of equipment that can assist with grooming. One such piece is a denture brush that suctions to the sink to assist with denture cleaning. Other pieces may be long-handled hairbrushes or combs to assist with reach to both sides of one's head. Another adaptation often made is for men to use electric razors. This is for several reasons: one, it is often easier to manage than a regular razor and shaving cream, and two, persons who have had a stroke are commonly taking blood thinners. If cutting oneself while shaving is a potential risk, an electric razor is certainly the best solution.

Bathing

One-handed techniques and simple adaptations may be used to increase one's independence in showering. Long-handled sponges can aid in reaching to one's feet and back more easily as well. Wrapping a washcloth around the shoulder of one's strong arm aids in washing it, as does placing the soaped cloth on one's knee and rubbing the strong arm along the leg. Crossing one's leg up over the knee may aid in being able to reach to one's feet without bending forward and risking falling over.

Bathing is an area where adaptation becomes essential for safety and increasing independence. One of the single most recommended pieces of equipment is a shower bench or a transfer tub bench. These benches may allow persons with stroke to bathe independently once they are seated. A caregiver does not have to worry about balance problems or weakness that would cause concerns if the person were to stand on a slippery surface.

There are many different kinds of benches, and selection depends on many things. The first decision to be made is whether or not the person will be able to step over the side of the bathtub. If so, a shower bench would be appropriate. Next is the question of whether skin integrity is a problem. If the person has fragile skin, a padded bench may be necessary. The degree to which one can hold one's balance and the level of fatigue one experiences during showering will determine the need for a back on the bench. The next decision is a financial one, since many insurance companies (including Medicare) do not cover bathtub-seating equipment. The cost of the bench may also be one of the determining factors in bench selection. Whatever the decision, the bench should be sturdy, be made of rust-free material, be adjustable for height, and preferably have flat bottomed, rubber-tipped feet. Along with benches, it is also recommended that the person with stroke obtain a hand-held showerhead to control direction of the water and protection from hot water surges that may occur and not be noticed due to delayed sensation.

Dressing

One of the more frustrating things about relearning after a stroke is relearning how to dress oneself. Many an individual has commented that living in a nudist colony would be easier than having to deal with one-handed dressing on a daily basis. The fact is that it is quite difficult to get dressed if one side of the body is considerably weaker. If one adds any other problems into the mix, it certainly makes this task a most challenging one.

Adapted dressing for the person who has had a stroke, often referred to as hemi-dressing technique, is important for the individual to perceive himself as independent and for maintaining dignity and self-image. This technique can be used for any kind of clothing, but generally loose fitting and flexible fabrics such as cotton make it much easier to perform. When dressing, the person with stroke should start by putting the weaker side in the garment first. When removing clothing, the person removes clothing on the weaker side last. The reason for this adaptation is that the weaker side cannot assist in getting the clothes on as well, so the maximum amount of maneuvering is performed by the side that is stronger. It is best for the individual to be seated and to not try to rush through dressing. It is easier to avoid mistakes than correct them later. Dressing equipment is not widely used with persons who have had strokes, primarily because it is difficult enough having to manage things with one hand, let alone adding a foreign object to help. The most likely adaptation is a long-handled shoehorn. However, those who are wearing an ankle-foot orthosis (AFO) can use the brace as a shoehorn for the weaker foot and that generally takes care of the problem. Other commonly used pieces of equipment are adaptations for shoe tying. There are a variety of devices to substitute for having to tie shoes: one is elastic shoelaces that are tied and left tied for the wearer to slip on and off. Velcro shoe fasteners are widely available on shoes for any age group. Another is shoe buttons that are inserted into the top hole of the shoe and then the laces are tied around the button-to untie the shoe, the wearer leaves the lace tied and unhooks it from around the button. These are two popular ways of adapting shoe tying. Lastly there is a technique for one-handed shoe tying that relies on good perceptual skills, re-lacing one's shoes, and cooperative caregivers not helping too much by retying the laces.

Functional Mobility

A person who has suffered a stroke may have difficulty moving the arm and leg, balancing in sitting or standing, and difficulty with coordination and sensation. This makes it difficult to move in bed (roll, come to a sitting position), come to a standing position, and complete a transfer. It is even more challenging to walk.

A transfer is the process of moving from one surface to another. Transfers can be done in many ways. If the person who has suffered a stroke can stand, he may be able to do a stand-pivot transfer. This type of transfer involves standing up from one surface and pivoting or turning so they can sit down on another surface. If standing is not possible, the transfer can be done in a squatting position, or with the use of a sliding board. A sliding board serves as a bridge between two surfaces (i.e., wheelchair and bed). The person sits on the board and slides from one surface to the other. All transfers generally require the assistance of a therapist or caregiver, until full independence is achieved.

Another functional mobility task that may be challenging for someone who has had with a stroke is moving the wheelchair. An unfamiliar task to most whom have suffered a stroke, propelling a wheelchair is a way of getting from one place to the other if walking is not possible. A therapist provides instructions on how to use a wheelchair. One way a wheelchair can be propelled is by using the strong arm and leg. In this case, the stronger arm pushes the large rear wheel on the wheelchair and the stronger foot, which is in contact with the floor, helps pull the chair forward. Another option is to use either both arms or both legs. The method used depends on the strength of the affected arm and leg.

Walking is perhaps the most challenging task facing people with stroke. In order to begin to walk, someone must be able to come to a standing position with or without help. He has to be able to keep his balance in a standing position. He must also be strong enough to begin to move the weak leg forward so as to take a step. Taking steps also requires significant trunk control and strength. Sometimes a person with stroke has difficulty activating or controlling the muscles in his foot or ankle. These are very important for walking. In this case an an-kle foot orthosis (AFO) may be used. Walkers and various types of canes are also used when the person with stroke begins to walk again. These devices help the person who has weakness in his leg and/or problems with balance and sensation. They may reduce the need for caregiver assistance.

More advanced walking skills are climbing up and down stairs/curbs, and walking on uneven surfaces. When a person with stroke learns to climb stairs it is best to use a rail and go up and down the stairs one step at a time. When going up the stairs, the strong leg al-ways steps up first followed by the weaker leg. When going down the stairs, the weaker leg goes down first and is followed by the strong leg. The same procedure is used to go up and down a curb. Walking on uneven terrain such as sidewalks, grass, and ramps requires good bal-ance and strength.

EQUIPMENT

Mobility

There are many pieces of equipment that can be of great use to the person with stroke. Among them are wheelchairs and wheelchair cushions/backs, assistive devices such as canes and walkers, and or-thotic devices.

Wheelchairs are often necessary as a means of getting around. Some with strokes may use the wheelchair temporarily until they are able to return to walking, while others may use the wheelchair indefi-nitely. In either situation, the wheelchair provides a safe and efficient means of mobility for the person who has had a stroke.

Wheelchairs come in various sizes and with many different options. A therapist will take measurements in a sitting position of the person who will use the wheelchair. These measurements will help decide the size and type of the wheelchair to be used. If the wheelchair user will be propelling the wheelchair with the stronger foot, it is important that the wheelchair height allow the user to reach the floor with one's foot.

Among the wheelchair options that should be considered when or-dering a wheelchair are wheel lock extensions and a seat belt. Wheel lock extensions are long tubes place on top of the wheel locks so as to make them easier to reach. They will allow the wheelchair user to reach over to his weaker side with his strong hand to lock the wheel.

This is necessary when the weak arm/hand is not strong enough to manipulate the wheel lock. A seat belt is an important positioning device and is easily mounted to the wheelchair frame. It is used both for safety as well as positioning.

The sitting position of the wheelchair user is very important. Many types of wheelchair cushions are available. They are made from many different materials. Some are meant for more full-time wheelchair users and help encourage an optimal seated position, and others are meant for people who use the wheelchair less frequently. For people who are using the wheelchair more often, a solid seat may be used underneath the wheelchair cushion. Attached by way of drop hooks to the frame of the wheelchair or as an insert into the wheelchair cushion, the solid seat is usually made of wood or a thick plastic material. It provides a solid base upon which a person can sit. Sitting on a solid base encourages good posture and proper positioning of the arms and legs.

Wheelchair back cushions are also utilized when optimal positioning is desired. These cushions are usually recommended for more full-time wheelchair users. They are made from many different materials, and in some cases can be adapted to meet the postural needs of the user. They are mounted onto the back of the wheelchair and often replace the sling upholstery in the wheelchair. Wheelchair back cushions are important to keep the trunk in a good position.

Another piece of equipment that may be added to a wheelchair is a lap tray. This piece of equipment is used to position the weaker arm and to protect the arm from being caught in the wheelchair parts. Usually, these trays are used when a person with stroke has little to no movement in one arm or has a very weak trunk. There are full lap trays, which extend from one arm of the wheelchair to the other, and there are half lap trays that attach to one arm of the wheelchair and extend across half of the person seated. There are benefits and limits to each type of lap tray. The therapists working with the patient can help determine which one may be most appropriate. Full lap trays provide support for not only the whole arm, but the upper body as well. These are especially beneficial when someone is very weak following a stroke. Another benefit is that there is always a working surface in front of the person seated in the chair. These trays may also be used on other chairs when the person is not sitting in the wheelchair. Half lap trays provide a little less support for the upper body but allow for better access in and out of the wheelchair. These trays are only used on wheelchairs, but they slide over the arm of the wheelchair to allow for easier transfer in

and out of the chair. If a wheelchair is only for the short term, it is recommended to find another strategy to position the weaker arm.

In many situations, it is initially impossible for the person with
stroke to move the foot or ankle. In other cases, the foot and ankle
may be very weak. In either case, the foot and ankle are in need of
support if walking is to be done safely and efficiently. A brace called
an ankle foot orthosis (AFO) can be used to support the foot. Use of
this brace ensures that the foot will clear the floor and not drag as the
person walks. The brace can be made out of plastic or metal. Plastic
braces are either prefabricated or custom molded depending on the
person's needs. They are worn inside a shoe. The metal braces can be
attached to the outside of a shoe.

Other important devices that can be used to make walking easier are
canes and walkers. There are many varieties of canes and walkers available. Canes most useful for the person who has suffered a stroke are
quad canes and single point canes. Four point quad canes have four
legs at the base and come in large-base and small-base sizes. Each cane
has four points attached to its base, which are in contact with the floor.
These canes are made of metal and are adjustable in height.

Someone who needs less support when walking may use a single
point cane. This cane provides the least support of all the canes. It
gives the user only a steadying assist while walking. These canes are
made of metal or wood. They can be adjustable and come with a variety of handgrips.

If a person with stroke has use of both arms/hands, a walker may be
used. There are many types of walkers available. All are made of metal
tubing and most are adjustable in height. Wheels can be added to the
front of the walker to allow for a smoother pattern of walking. As with
the quad canes, the walker has four points in contact with the floor.
Because of this and its wider base of support, it gives the user a lot of
stability when walking.

Splinting

Often after a stroke, there is weakness or loss of sensation or coordination in one arm. There is a wide range in the amount that one will
be able to use his arm after a stroke, and changes in abilities to use
one's hand and arm can be seen for up to a year following stroke recovery. One should remember when going through the rehabilitation
process that there are very few people with stroke who are able to use

their weaker arm exactly as they did before the stroke. Usually, immediately after a stroke, there is severe weakness with or without changes in sensation. During this period of weakness, one should be monitoring the position of one's arm and hand constantly to make sure it is not under his body, hanging from the bed, or in any other compromising or dangerous position. At this stage it may be determined that a splint is needed to maintain the position of the hand. Resting hand splints are commonly given to support the arches of the hand and to protect the hand from being positioned where damage could occur to the joints or overstretching could occur in the muscles and tendons. These splints are typically worn at night, though they may be worn during the day, too. There is usually a schedule for wear, and the user should check for areas or pressure or points of discomfort each time the splint is removed. The splint should be checked periodically for proper fit as well.

In cases where the hand muscles seem to be working but weak and the arm is starting to move but there is weakness along the arm, a wrist splint may or may not be provided to support a weak wrist and allow finger movement. A wrist splint may be provided in cases where the muscles that extend the wrist are weak, but there is movement in other parts of the arm. Many times this splint is provided to assist hand function and worn until the wrist muscles are strong enough to do the work for themselves during daily tasks.

Toileting

Another area of concern for individuals recovering from stroke is the ability to use the toilet independently. Problems with balance and sensation as well as difficulty with self-monitoring can interfere with someone safely completing his toileting alone.

There are several different parts to this task, the first being the ability to get on and off of the toilet. One takes for granted that he or she can get up and down readily from one of these seats, as they are quite low. For the individual who may have trouble with balance or weakness in the trunk or one leg, lowering oneself down to the toilet is challenging. The first thing the occupational therapist looks at is equipment that raises the height of the seat to a manageable level. This varies, so something adjustable, like a commode chair or a three-in-one-commode is a good choice. This device gets its name from its features: it can be used next to the bed for someone who is not mobile, it can raise the height of the toilet, and it can be used as grab bars or safety rails around the toilet to make lowering and raising easier.

Another piece of related equipment is a raised toilet seat, preferably one with handles. This seat clamps onto any toilet and is thus a more portable option for someone who visits family members often and wants to be able to take along the equipment. Another, less cumbersome piece of equipment is a toilet safety rail that attaches to the bolts on the toilet seat and wraps around the toilet without raising the height of the seat. This equipment is usually for someone who may need a bit of balancing help or a boost off of the low seat.

The next part of the toileting task that becomes difficult is managing clothing before and after. It is difficult to manage fasteners and openings in a timely manner when time may be short. Furthermore, it may be one-handed technique that one is using while trying to balance on one weak leg and one strong one. Many individuals prefer elastic waist bands or drawstring style pants that make pants management easier. Pants that fasten with velcro are also available at some stores.

The last part of this task that may be problematic is cleaning oneself after toileting. For some individuals, this is essential to maintain dignity, yet it may be difficult to balance while reaching behind to clean. There are some alternatives available. One is a sitz bath type of cleaning system, similar to a bidet that clasps around the toilet rim. If a person's size is what is limiting, there are toilet tissue holders that have handles on them to aid in reaching behind to clean. Discussion of these options may be difficult but important to preserve a sense of privacy and dignity for the newly disabled person.

Cooking

Many persons with stroke want to be able to get their own meals when they return home from the hospital. If it is not possible to use both hands, it is still possible to be able to get things done in the kitchen with some minor pieces of equipment. There are adapted cutting boards that make it possible to cut with one hand. These boards have two rust proof nails that stick up through the board to stabilize what is being cut. These boards also have raised edges that make it easier to spread things on bread when making sandwiches.

One of the toughest things about working in some kitchens after a stroke is carrying things with one hand and managing a cane or a walker. Often, the one hand that a person has left to help with things is using a cane and that makes moving around quite difficult. It is sometimes a recommendation to buy a rolling cart that makes carrying things easier. Another recommendation, depending on how far things need to be carried, is to slide them along the counter from one place to another. It may be possible to rearrange things in the kitchen to make it easier to gather needed items so they do not need to be carried. Another solution is to use an apron with pockets and Tupperware or bottles to carry things if the distance is far. There are many creative options that can help solve these problems. Some people just bring a stool into the kitchen and clear off a spot for eating at the counter. Then there is no need to carry the food once it is ready.

Housekeeping

Many people do not plan to do light housekeeping at home after a stroke, and it is recommended that a person take it easy for a while during his recovery. If one is planning to return to these activities right away, it is important to set aside a part of the day for rest following cleaning in order to conserve energy. There are many important strategies for energy conservation. One strategy is to do things while sitting down as much as possible. Tasks such as emptying the dishwasher, vacuuming, bed making, and dusting or cooking are not only less energy draining if done while seated, but also are safer for most people with weakness or problems with balance. Spending thirty minutes dusting should be followed by at least thirty minutes of rest to regain strength and energy.

Housekeeping tasks should be done on days when not much else is planned so that the energy used is focused toward those activities. They should also be done at times during the day when energy levels are higher, such as the morning. A person with stroke is more likely to lose his balance or trip over things more when tired. Another important energy conservation strategy is to be aware of how tired one feels before starting a chore and during a chore. If it is possible, when getting tired stop in order to save energy. Try not to plan too much for one session and allow breaks or even finish the task another day if necessary.

Driving

Driving is a very complex task involving many physical, sensory, cognitive, and visual skills. Thus, there are many challenges involved in returning to driving after one has had a stroke. Two of the primary things that are addressed by the therapist are vision and cognition. These are difficult problems to measure and are sometimes harder for individuals or family members to understand. If a person has lost some of his visual field as a result of the stroke, the first thing to do is to have the extent of that loss measured to determine whether there is enough remaining vision to allow the person with stroke to drive legally. Each state has different motor vehicle requirements, but a therapist trained in driving rehabilitation or a local licensing agency should be able to provide that information. A person with visual perceptual problems or neglect should most likely not drive because of the dangers posed to one's self and others.

If a person's cognition is impaired, anticipating the actions of other drivers may be difficult. Reaction times to events around him may be slowed, or he may have difficulty attending to all of the things necessary for driving. A person needs to be able to attend to many things at once in order to return to driving. A driver-training therapist may look at the places a person drove before the stroke, around the neighborhood or to the doctor, and determine that the person may be safe for those familiar places. The therapist may recommend that someone else do the driving on longer trips, or in unfamiliar places.

If a person with stroke has paralysis or weakness in the right leg, the driver-training therapist will examine how effectively the person can use the accelerator and the brake and how efficiently this is done. If someone has poor sensation of where the right leg is in space, chances are good that equipment recommendations will be made. Left foot accelerators are commonly recommended for someone with right-sided weakness. This equipment is attached to the floor of the car and is used with the car brake in the same way a typical gas pedal is used. It is a safe way to use the left foot to drive.

If a person has weakness in either arm following a stroke, a spinner knob is usually recommended to help with turning the wheel completely. These knobs fit over the steering wheel and make turning the wheel easier with one hand. There are also attachments to extend the controls of the car so they may be located on the left side in the case of right arm weakness. Anyone with any weakness should have access to an automatic shift car with power brakes and steering. Any equipment that is obtained should be reported to the local licensing agency to inform them of the reasons for its use so that it may be noted.

Lastly, it is generally up to a person's doctor to determine when it is safe to return to driving. Consult with the physician about plans to return to driving and when that may be possible. A reasonable time frame is anywhere between three months to a year after a stroke.

Finances

Managing money can be difficult for anyone at times, but it can be especially after stroke. The person may have language and numeric difficulty. Sometimes these individuals cannot recognize amounts of money or numbers. Then someone else needs to be responsible for the finances. Other times, adding and subtracting the numbers in one's head is difficult, and there is a need to use other strategies. Money is an area where other people can easily take advantage of the person with stroke. It is a good idea to know how much one can handle before going into money-management situations. It is a good idea to establish the meaning of different amounts of money, if one is able to recognize a price and provide that amount of money, and to be able to determine if there is enough money to purchase the items. These are strategies for day-to-day purchases. Budgeting and checkbook management are also areas to address with someone with difficulty with numbers or with cognitive problems as a result of his stroke. Using strategies to pay attention to details and make sure total amounts of items have been addressed are important for these individuals. Stroke survivors learn to double-check themselves for accuracy of calculations and omissions. Sometimes it is less frustrating for the individual and family members for someone else to take over the bookkeeping. However, this is usually a significant loss of a role for the person with stroke. Perhaps some part of the responsibility can be shared or done jointly to keep the person involved.

The stroke survivor's physical and cognitive skills and capacities will improve in the weeks and months following the stroke. As a result the person will become progressively more independent in all areas of daily living and mobility. They will adapt their abilities as the demands of the environment change. The combined efforts of the stroke survivor and the rehabilitation team will provide clear understanding of how the person was affected by the stroke and what therapeutic interventions and equipment will benefit the person most in the return to a satisfying, enjoyable life.

Table 8.1 Making a Plan for Myself

1. What are my problems?

The answers to the question and the problems are yours to describe. The problem you may have depends on your own particular situation and your concerns.

1. _____
2. _____
3. _____

The answers to the question of goals are also yours to describe. It is helpful not only to specify what you wish to accomplish, but how much, or how fast, or how independently. When answering the question about what results you find have been achieved, it is helpful to specify not only what the results were but where or when it happened. The answers to the question about what works may also be your ideas or equipment you have found useful. It is helpful not only to specify what you do to contribute to the results, but how you go about it. "How often" or "where" or "when" are some additional questions to help make your statements more specific.

2. Following my plan

Participation: Agreement (A) Confirmed Agreement (CA) Statement (S) Specific Statement (SS)			
Date	**Status/Progress**	**Goals**	**What Works**
	☐	☐	☐
	☐	☐	☐
	☐	☐	☐
	☐	☐	☐

9

Quality of Life After Stroke

F. CAROL BULLARD-BATES
HELEN BOZZO
JENNIFER DAVIES HENDRICKS

Stroke is an event that affects you and your family's mind, body, and soul. In this chapter, you will learn about psychosocial and emotional issues that occur as a direct result of damage to a specific part of the brain. You will also be introduced to many of the resources in the community, including home health care, that can assist you during your transition back into the community. The end of this chapter (Table 9.1) contains a log for the patient with stroke to write down the goals, problems, questions, and successes that are experienced when striking back at stroke.

PSYCHOSOCIAL AND EMOTIONAL ISSUES

The challenges you face after a stroke affect all areas of your life. In this chapter we discuss the changes that may occur after stroke in your emotional, social, spiritual, language, thinking/perception/memory functioning, as well as changes that may occur in your family interactions. Since stress management is essential if you are to regain your health and emotional stability, we suggest lifestyle changes and techniques to maintain a calm state of mind and a healthy body. Another issue is how to deal with pain if this is a problem after your stroke.

Finally we describe the role of the social worker or case manager in your recovery and rehabilitation, the different levels of rehabilitation available after you leave the acute care hospital, the important issues to be aware of in your rehabilitation program and in your discharge planning, and the community resources you may need after returning home. Home care nursing and therapy support are described, as are the important issues to be aware of in your plan for this phase of your recovery. We hope that this information will enhance the quality of your and your family's life as you support each other in identifying and solving the problems that you face after stroke.

The very word "stroke" gives one a sense of the drastic change it can bring in one's life. I remember my fears when my husband had taken a friend of ours to the Mayo Clinic for diagnostic tests and he ended up in the hospital with a stroke himself. A call I made to him was devastating to me. His speech was slowed as he told me the story of being in a restaurant and realizing he could not read the menu or see on the right. As I asked him questions about the doctor's comments, I realized his memory was poor. Then I asked him to get a pencil and write down my questions for the doctor. After we had painstakingly gone through the process of him writing and I asked him to read me what I had said, he could not do so.

Months later, he had regained his strength to some degree and was driving again, he went to "cheer up" his 90-year-old mother in Cincinnati. While they were driving, he missed seeing a car that was illegally parked on the side of the road. The accident injured his mother to the degree that we questioned whether she would survive the ordeal. He never drove again. Reading, one of the loves of his life, was an incredible chore. It took him four to five times longer than it had before the stroke. All this happened with what many professionals would call a "mini-stroke".

Brain Attack: The Emotional Front

A stroke attacks us at the very heart of our entire being: our brain, the organ that defines our identity and our experience as human beings and allows us to interact in our world smoothly and easily. Even small changes in this organ, then, can disrupt our lives in powerful ways. The emotional changes in you and your loved ones after a stroke, therefore, are not surprising. Depression is the most common and is not unexpected considering the many losses you may suffer after a stroke: loss of strength, control of movement, sensation, vision, speech, swallowing, comprehension, clarity and speed of thinking, attention, memory, visual perception, planning and organizing. These losses often result in periods of grief and sadness as you face the changes they bring. As in any grief process, there may be periods of shock, denial, anger, or bitterness as you discover the extent of your challenges at each phase of your recovery. It is important to be aware of the signs of when a normal grief process has become serious clinical depression, however, and needs medication and psychotherapy to enable you to regain your emotional equilibrium. This needs to be watched for in those of you who have suffered significant depression before your stroke or if you have had parents or siblings with a history of depression. The symptoms of a clinical depression include problems with your sleep pattern, such as either not being able to get to sleep, frequent awakening during the night, early morning awakening, or sleeping too much during the day.

Appetite changes are frequent. Often the person with stroke has a poor appetite; sometimes he eats too much. The feeling of not caring about much in your life, or the loss of energy or motivation to get up and face the day can be another sign of depression. When this turns into a desire to die or thoughts of death, or methods of how you might kill yourself, then you or your loved one are suffering from a serious degree of depression needing immediate treatment. You and your family need to take any suicidal comments, even if presented in a joking format, very seriously. It may be difficult to discuss these issues with each other, but it is essential to avoid the tragedy of a life snuffed out too early because of a treatable depression.

Other symptoms of depression include fatigue, irritability, frequent crying spells, disinterest in things that you usually enjoyed, disinterest in sex, desire for isolation from your friends or family, and a sense of hopelessness and helplessness. If these symptoms have been problems over several weeks, you need to consider getting help. Going to your general practitioner can be a first step, although some doctors tend to give people tranquilizers (e.g.,Valium) for depression.These can cause even more problems. Ask your doctor for antidepressant medication, preferably a serotonin reuptake inhibitor that can give you new physical and emotional energy and allow you to feel "yourself" again. If your general practitioner is not comfortable in prescribing this type of medication, ask him or her for a referral to a psychiatrist whom he or she respects and works with regularly. There are other antidepressant medications helpful with serious sleep problems (e.g.,Sinequan, Elavil). Most of these medications take up to three or four weeks to fully take effect, so do not despair if the effect is not immediate.

Fear, anxiety and worry are other common problems after a stroke, and have many issues causing them to be maintained. "Will I have another stroke?" "Will I recover from this stroke?" "Will my blood pressure/blood sugar stay uncontrolled?" "Will my wife/husband/partner still love me with this stroke?" "Will we make it financially if I can not go back to work?" Whatever the answers are to these questions, they may still linger in your mind. They may raise their ugly heads when you may be feeling particularly tired or discouraged. I recommend that you do two things when these emotions threaten to overwhelm you. Ask yourself the question, "Am I doing everything I can do to keep myself healthy, to love my family, and to get back to work?" If you feel you are, then congratulate yourself and develop a list of enjoyable things to distract yourself from your fears and worries when they arise. These may include relaxation exercises, reading, listening to music, doing a new hobby (see the stress management section below). If you recognize that you can make improvements in some of the areas of concern, then develop your own list of goals. At the conclusion of this chapter is a work sheet to list your problems and action plans/goals to solve these problems. Examples of goals you might set toward a path of wellness are as follows: "I will no longer go to McDonald's for a quick hamburger and french fries" "I will say something appreciative to my husband for the things he does for me every day" "I will talk to a colleague who will keep our conversation confidential and to my therapists/doctor about the things necessary to go back to work". Fear, worry, and anxiety cause us to lose our energy and drain our emotional reserves. If you are able to attack your worries with a positive, constructive approach, then you can regain your motivation to live the best possible life. A small amount of anxiety in many situations can be helpful for you to mobilize your resources and do something about a difficult or challenging situation. Yet some of you have been worriers from childhood and may have had problems with fear and anxiety overwhelming you for many years. If you feel this is the case, and your stroke or the stroke of your loved one has made things much worse, you need to consider seeing a psychiatrist for possible medication. You should consider psychotherapy with a mental health professional, a psychologist, social worker, or your minister or rabbi.

Phobias

Although rare, phobias can occur after a stroke and are expressed usually with a phobic reaction to walking or climbing or descending stairs.

You may feel overwhelmed by the fear of falling. This reaction essentially can emotionally paralyze you as you attempt to move, even though you are physically capable of safely handling the action. Teaching yourself to relax before you attempt the action of your phobia is the first step. Then, maintain a relaxed state as you imagine yourself in your mind's eye performing the action comfortably and smoothly. Imagine how each limb goes through the necessary movement and how each movement feels. If you begin to become tense and scared while imagining this, stop the image of yourself moving and return to a relaxed state again before continuing.

Once you are able to maintain a relaxed state with the image of yourself making the needed movements, actually begin the action with a loved one close at hand. If your emotions get out of control again, stop the movements, stand still or sit down, and take the time needed to become relaxed again. If you have trouble in overcoming the phobia successfully, it is important to find a psychologist who will work with you to overcome it. The longer the phobia lasts, the more difficult it is to overcome. Getting help sooner rather than later is important.

Frustration, Anger, Irritability, and Poor Self-Control

Even those who have always been easygoing and relaxed in their lives before their stroke may find themselves easily irritated, upset, and angry after. A stroke causes you to have to depend on others for many simple things, and to have to figure out new ways of doing things. It may result in large amounts of time in accomplishing even the most minor activities in your life. No wonder then that the majority of persons with stroke end up easily frustrated by such everyday tasks as getting the toothpaste top off the tube, putting a shirt on, or opening a milk container. A one handed life is a constant hassle. For those of you with trouble with your temper before the stroke, the problem can be devastating for your relationships with your loved ones. For it is always they, those who are closest to you and who are doing their best to help you, that receive the brunt of your anger. This anger can even lead to physical and emotional abuse that will drive your loved ones away very quickly To better control your anger and irritability, try to follow these simple steps:

Be aware of the signs of when your anger or irritability is building.

- Perhaps you start to feel warm, your muscles tense, and your heart starts beating faster.
- If you are doing something that is getting you angry, stop what you are doing and take a break
- Take a deep breath, and as you breathe out, try to relax your body until those symptoms start to disappear.
- Ask yourself what was making you irritable or angry and what you can do to help the situation.

Cutting off that build up of anger is essential if you are going to stay healthy and your relationships are to remain stable. If you have trouble controlling your anger with these techniques, try seeing a mental health professional for some help. Couple or family sessions as well as individual sessions may be important to see the pattern of the problem and to help each person make needed changes to defuse the situation.

Poor Self Esteem and Self Image

The blow of a stroke to your image of yourself and your identity can not be underestimated. We are all controlled by the media and the images of beauty only attainable by a small percentage of our population. In our American culture, significant value is placed on independence. We have a certain image of ourselves in which is contained our physical attractiveness, our personality characteristics, our accomplishments, our roles in our families, our work, play, and prayer. All of these can be drastically changed at the moment of suffering a stroke. Many patients have shared with me their feelings of almost being like a baby again, having to learn how to control their urine and bowel movements, how to walk, how to speak, how to write, and how to get dressed. Being initially dependent on others is one of the most difficult things to cope with, particularly in the areas of toileting and bathing with its loss of privacy. The change in your looks can be shocking. Sometimes you see in the mirror that half of your face has dropped and your smile is only half expressing what you want to convey. Or perhaps your face has lost its former bright expression and is now always flat and lifeless. The energy and enthusiasm in your life may seem a distant image as you trudge through each day waiting for help with each basic function. Your family may have taken over the activities that you felt were so precious to you at home. You can no longer be the reader, the mechanic, the cook, the secretary, the gardener, the church elder, or the construction worker that defined you as a person before your stroke. So who are you now? The sooner you begin to grapple with that question with yourself and your loved ones, the better you will be able to weather the early stages of your recovery. Each phase of recovery may bring a different answer. Ask yourself "What are the most important things to me in my life and what can I do now? What are my goals, my problems?" Refer to the log at the end of this chapter to figure out what your questions are. No matter what your physical, thinking or speech limitations are, you can still show love to those whom you love. A smile and a squeeze of the hand is precious to each of us. You can still enjoy music and time with family members and friends. If we have love and share it, we remain our essential self, no matter how we express it. You will continue to recover many of the things that were precious to you, and those you do not will seem less essential as time goes on. Acceptance of the stroke may never fully come, but be open to new avenues of defining yourself. See each new accomplishment with pride and confidence, no matter how small. The various stories of stroke survivors ("Consumers Speak Out") in Part IV of this text will provide ample evidence of the indomitable human spirit. You will read about recovery from stroke against large odds and coping with disability that is at once heroic and fairly common among "strokers".

Emotional Lability

One rather odd consequence of a stroke may be a problem with not being able to control your laughing or crying. Our brains allow us to control our emotions most of the time when we are sad or happy, and to express certain feelings at appropriate times and with appropriate people. However, after a stroke you may lose this ability. You may find yourself crying uncontrollably when you are not sad during a visit from a friend or family member. You may laugh at inappropriate times, such as when someone is telling you about a sad event. Explaining the problem to your friends and family is important so they will not think you are constantly depressed or are being thoughtless of their issues or feelings. You may be able to control this by thinking of something peaceful or calm. Try just staring at your hand or an object in the room to distract yourself. A patient once described this unusual experience by stating that "I'm depressed because I am crying, I'm not crying because I'm depressed."

Personality Changes after a Stroke

Your personality traits may be exaggerated after a stroke. If you tend to be an obsessive- compulsive or an overcontrolling person, this characteristic may become worse. This can be very problematic for you and your loved ones, since they will have difficulty accomplishing things in your manner. You may have extreme difficulty with having others do things for you. This may represent too much loss of control over your life. Perhaps you will put yourself and your health or safety at risk if you do things you are not ready to do yet. Learning to accept help graciously is an important step and represents character strength in you, just as learning to become independent again does.

   In contrast, you may be a more passive person, and one who easily allows others to tell you what to do, say, or feel rather than standing up for yourself. A stroke may make you feel even more passive and help-less, and it may be tempting to allow others to do things for you that you have learned to do for yourself. It is faster or easier for some peo-ple. You might consider a goal of telling your family what you have learned to do already. Then their actions will not unknowingly create more dependency in you. Your log (see the log at the end of this chap-ter) will help you document your goals and achievement.

Emotional/Behavioral Changes after a Right Hemisphere Stroke with Left Sided Weakness

Poor awareness of the changes in your life since your right hemi-sphere stroke is most challenging in your recovery process early on. I have treated people with a right hemisphere stroke. They tell me that they are moving their left arm when they are not, or tell their family that they have been walking that day when they had not walked since their stroke. The degree of this poor self awareness seems to be re-lated to the degree of attention one is able to pay to the left side of your body and space. It is what we call left sided attention. It appears that the right hemisphere controls your ability to pay attention to your left side, and if you can not do this well, you are not aware of how weak you are or how that weakness has affected your life. We call this left inattention, or neglect. It may be seen in all three sensory avenues: what you see, what you feel and what you hear. It may be more evident in only one or two of your senses.

Because of this problem of poor awareness, you are more likely to have accidents. You think you can do things by yourself when you are not safe to do so. Many professionals have described people with right hemisphere strokes as impulsive. This means you are not able to control the speed at which you behave, in spite of repeated reminders to do so. You may be impulsive in thought and action. Much of this problem can be attributed to your problems with self awareness. If you do not perceive there is any real problem, why would you have to slow down and do things carefully? Many of us may move quickly before a stroke and tend to continue to do so afterwards unless we experience some sense of a change in our abilities. Because of this lack of awareness, you may not feel a sense of depression or loss as soon as others after a stroke. But as awareness improves, the feelings of loss are more evident and may cause more depression and worry.

Although rare, you can have problems with visual hallucinations after a right hemisphere stroke. Usually the hallucinations occur with significant problems with visual spatial processing and neglect. The hallucinations are not usually frightening as they may be with schizophrenic patients. One of my patients saw cigarettes everywhere, especially in patterns on long, oblong curtains and walls. He was trying to quit smoking. Another patient saw mice and spiders everywhere, but was not upset by these perceptions. This patient also had another problem that occurs infrequently, again usually with severe left neglect and poor visual spatial processing. He misperceived people in the hospital as people he thought were friends and relatives. He discussed this problem with me after several instances in which he approached a few people as his relatives. He discovered they did not know him. He and I developed a technique in which he would approach the person he thought he recognized, and if he or she did not say hello or appear to recognize him, he would assume that his mind was "playing tricks" on him. Reminding yourself that these experiences are from your stroke and doing a reality check with hospital staff or your family at home is helpful . It is possible that your mind will play tricks on you after a right hemisphere stroke, and it is important that you ask those around you for support and reality checks. If the experiences are very upsetting, a psychiatrist can be helpful in prescribing medication to reduce the hallucinations, and a mental health professional can provide support and reassurance, as well as help you with ways of coping with these changes.

Emotional/Behavioral Changes after Left Hemisphere Stroke

The emotional reactions after a left frontal hemisphere stroke are strikingly different from a left posterior stroke. After a left frontal hemisphere stroke, you will have significant weakness of the right side of your body, relatively good comprehension , but will have challenges in expressing yourself well, often being unable to do so, or only being able to say single words or phrases. This tends to lead to early problems with frustration and depression, even to the point of what has been called a "catastrophic reaction," in which you feel trapped, desperate, depressed, and tend to give up in trying to respond at times. Your problems with speech are all too obvious to you, and you are faced with a constant need in interactions with hospital staff and family members to use a faculty that you have essentially lost to make your needs known. Often you also face the problem with loss of motor sequences as you attempt to use your strong left arm and hand to perform tasks you want to accomplish, or in making your needs known nonverbally with gestures, or your tone of voice. This can lead to further frustration and tension. You may lash out at family members for their inability to understand what you are trying to communicate. This can occur in spite of their ardent attempts to guess what you are saying. As you become more tense and upset, your ability to communicate deteriorates. I constantly remind my patients with these challenges to "take a deep breath and try to calm down" in the midst of their frustration. The more the distress increases, the poorer becomes their communication. Because you are very aware of your physical limitations, you will have the tendency to be more fearful and cautious in your therapy. This may also affect your progress. Whereas the person with a right brain stroke may have become "impulsive," the person with left brain stroke can be abnormally cautious or hesitant. You will be all too aware of your inability to move safely by yourself, and will therefore not tend to have as many accidents in the hospital or at home. You may have more difficulty trying new things because you might feel at risk of falling. This fear will definitely interfere with your progress. Learning to relax yourself before transferring from your bed to your wheelchair or before walking will help, as well as developing trust in your therapists or in your family members. They can keep you safe as you try each new activity. The encouraging fact about a stroke affecting the left frontal portion of the brain is that the person generally has excellent self awareness and good listening comprehension.

The emotional reactions after a posterior left hemisphere (towards the back of the brain) stroke are remarkably different and demonstrate a different pattern of language function. I will discuss only those people suffering a pattern of poor comprehension and fluent but meaningless speech after a posterior left hemisphere stroke. This is often called Wernicke's aphasia. With this pattern, all areas of language are severely affected, but movement is often relatively intact. What is striking about the person with this pattern is his or her initial lack of awareness of any problems whatsoever. I may ask the patient a question, and the patient will respond comfortably and easily and often at length, but what is said makes little sense and worse still, the patient is generally unaware of this fact. Although initially a person with these problems will seem unconcerned about this communication pattern, the "Wernicke's patient" later may develop frustration because he is asking people to do things and they are not following through. This may turn into a feeling of even greater frustration. The person may eventually feel isolated and paranoid since others appear to be ignoring him and his wishes. He still does not recognize the problem in his own communication pattern. Only when the person with Wernicke's aphasia recognizes problems with his own speech is there hope that he will begin to learn to make sense again. Unfortunately, sometimes word recovery does not occur.

Emotional Reactions after Frontal Lobe Stroke

We call the functions that the frontal lobes take care of as "executive functions." This is because these involve the kinds of things one needs to do as an executive in an office. These include the following functions:

- mental flexibility
- attention to and being able to handle two things at once
- organization and planning ahead
- initiation and sequencing of activities
- ending activities when needed
- completion of activities quickly and efficiently
- emotional control to respond in an emotionally appropriate way

There are two emotional reactions described in the literature after frontal lobe stroke. These depend on the area of the frontal lobe affected. Both emotional patterns can also be seen after brain injuries from accidents, since the frontal lobe is usually affected by trauma to the brain also. One pattern may make a person appear unemotional (described for right hemisphere stroke patients earlier) with little or no reaction to others or your environment. This does not mean you are not feeling things inside, but that there is no emotional facial reaction. Many people may misinterpret your flat face as depression, but this is usually not the case. Here again it is important for you to tell your family your feelings, since they will not be evident on your face or in your tone of voice. It may be difficult for you to initiate activities, and your responses may be slow. It may be difficult for you to sequence activities well, and you may have problems switching from one activity to another. You may get stuck on an action or thought sequence when it is no longer appropriate. This problem we call perseveration. Your attention is often poor, and also you may have a tendency to be forgetful and to lose track of what you were saying. Because your organization and memory can be poor, it is important to try to write out plans for the day and organize activities so you do not forget to accomplish the most important things. Many people with frontal lobe strokes can be seen as unmotivated because they do not initiate things quickly and will often be content to do relatively little unless others encourage them to be active.

The second pattern of emotional response is one characterized by disinhibited behavior and speech. Your emotional reactions may be out of control, and you may say what is on your mind, even if it is rude or a sexual come-on to someone not even known. Your behavior may demonstrate no regard for the thinking or feeling of others. It is hard for you to put yourself in someone else's place and have empathy or understanding for them. You may not be aware of the social mistakes you are making. One of my patients with frontal lobe damage after an aneurysm had been clipped (a ballooning wall of an artery) would walk down the street with his wife and reach out to women passing by and grab their breasts. This was done with inappropriate sexual comments as he did so. He was also sexually disinhibited with his wife, and wanted to have sex with her many times a day. He did not understand why she would be upset about this behavior. It was necessary to develop a behavioral contract between him and his wife specifying how often was reasonable for them to have sex. They kept a chart of sexual activity because he often did not have satisfactory recall of what had happened. We also listed behaviors that were appropriate and those that were not. His wife tried to accompany him or have someone else go with him on his walks to ensure he would not get in trouble with those not understanding his problem.

Emotional Responses after Brain Stem Stroke

Some of the most emotionally traumatic symptoms can occur with a brain stem stroke, such as dizziness, slurred speech, double vision, as well as weakness. These can be extremely overwhelming and disorienting problems. When dizziness is worse with head turning or movement, many stay still most of the time to avoid any more sense of loss of control. Focusing on relaxation of your muscles as you breathe out and keeping a peaceful scene in your mind can be helpful in attaining a greater feeling of control.

Emotional Responses after Corpus Callosum Stroke

This type of stroke is unusual in that it hits the nerve fibers in the brain connecting your right and left half of your brain. The emotional experience is extremely strange. You may perceive that your mind has lost conscious control of the left side of your body and is working against what you want to be doing. One of my patients reported that often when she was trying to get dressed in the morning, she would find her left hand unbuttoning her blouse as quickly as her right hand was buttoning it. This "alien hand" syndrome can be upsetting. Everything is more difficult to accomplish because your left hand either works against you or does something not related to what you are trying to do. My patient with this problem would have her left hand grasp the chair arm before she started an activity. This would sometimes keep her hand from working against her for a little longer. She experienced this as having another person inside her who was trying to exist and act separately from her own wishes. In fact, it was her own right hemisphere that was essentially no longer under her left hemisphere's conscious control. Since the right hemisphere appears to be more emotionally based, her left side would often surprise her with its emotional reactions, such as grabbing another piece of cake when she was trying to control her temptation to eat too much.

Spiritual Issues

For those who have a sense of God's presence in their lives, spiritual questions are often asked after a stroke. "Why did God allow this to happen to me? Is God punishing me for something I did in the past?" Rabbi Kushner's best selling book *When Bad Things Happen to Good People* might be very helpful for the patient who feels unfairly singled out by "an act of God." You may experience increased guilt over a perception of past sins for which you have not yet fully forgiven yourself. You may question your relationship with God or be angry at God for allowing your stroke to occur. You may wonder why God has not healed you fully when so many friends and family members have been praying for you. These feelings and questions are part of your spiritual journey and growth and need to be dealt with openly and honestly with those who will understand and with God. Most rehabilitation hospitals provide pastoral care services, and you would be well advised to use this religious resource if you are feeling spiritual challenges.

Family Communication

The stress on the family communication pattern after a stroke cannot be underestimated. Sharing your feelings in whatever way possible enables you to cope better with the drastic changes occurring in your lifestyle. Initially, very often your closest relationships can be controlled by what you may need physically, with your spouse or children being your caretakers rather than the friends they had been before. If tensions existed between family members before your stroke, these may be magnified by the stress you and your loved ones experience with your new limitations. There will be changes in responsibilities and demands on all those close to you. It is extremely important to ask your loved ones how they are coping. They are not only giving you the support you need, but also trying to keep the house running and other family members supported as well as being the communication center for the rest of your family and friends on your progress. Depression, anxiety, worry, fear, and exhaustion are all part of their experience too, as they try to balance their responsibilities and attempt to set up your home and your needed support network in the initial phases of your recovery. Ask your family members how you can help them in this balancing act.

Since this is probably one of the biggest crises ever to happen in your family, it is important for you to make sure each member of the family is getting the support and love they need. This is especially true if you have children in the home, whatever their age. The children who are acting out may be the ones you focus on, but it is often the quiet and noncommunicative child who needs the attention, but who gets the least. Having a mother or father suffer a stroke is extremely devastating to a child whose self-image is being formed. It is difficult for a child to have you look different and not to be able to play the roles with them as before. They, too, suffer a great deal of loss of support and activity as your spouse now needs to be your caretaker as well as theirs. This is especially true if you are a single parent. The love you and your spouse or other family members express to them is essential in helping them to recognize that they are still loved and cared for in spite of the changes in your family's lifestyle. Children often do more poorly in school after a family medical crisis such as a stroke, and it is important to make their teachers aware of the problem. Then the teachers can provide an understanding word or can encourage the child to share some of his/her feelings at recess or after school. This enables the child to feel less isolated or overwhelmed at school. If your child appears more angry, depressed, or irritable and does not seem to be eating or sleeping well at night over several weeks, you might ask the school counselor to talk to him. You might even consider calling in a mental health professional. Family meetings/evenings can also be helpful to discuss what everyone in the family is thinking or feeling and how developing problems can be resolved.

Role reversals in the family are particularly difficult after a stroke. Usually you may have done all the finances, but now your spouse, child, or other family member may have to take over. This may be very difficult for you to accept, and you may be uncomfortable with someone else doing a task that you had under good control. You may find that your children/family members are tending to make decisions without your input or consent. Be open about your feelings and ask each family member to keep you informed of the financial or other decisions they need to make. It is easy for you to feel more isolated from the family interactions, particularly when you suffer problems with speech, but it is essential to feel you are included at the level that you can participate in important family matters.

Setting up a Support System

One of the most important things I tell people who have just suffered a stroke is to accept help whenever it is offered. From the beginning of your stroke, family or friends will say "How can I help?" Accept these offers whenever they are made by figuring out what will be helpful for you in the next several weeks. We are often too oriented to being independent and do not rely on those outside our immediate family. And yet, many of us live at a distance from other family members. Then we cannot receive the needed support. Asking a friend to call before he goes to the grocery store to see if you need a few things can be an enormous help. Or setting up a schedule of friends to take turns taking you to therapy can give your spouse or child a break. Just having a list of people in the neighborhood to spend a few hours visiting with you when your loved one does something he/she enjoys can be a special gift to you both. It may be difficult for your pride actually to ask for this help. If you do it early in your recovery, however, it can be a blessing to have developed a network of supportive people that remains over the years.

Sexual Functioning

Sexual functioning can be significantly affected following a stroke, and many couples are less sexually active after a stroke. You may have less interest in sex (libido). Men may have more trouble maintaining erections and having ejaculations, and women may have more difficulty having orgasms. When one considers the many problems post stroke that can affect your sexual functioning, this is not surprising. It is more difficult for you to move, and positions you may have used for intercourse before may not be possible any more. You may have lost feeling in your affected side, and it is difficult to feel or be touched on that side. Pain can be a problem with your shoulder or other joints. This can interfere with your natural sexual responsiveness. You may be too exhausted by the end of the day to think of anything but going to sleep, when you were used to making love in the evenings before your stroke. You may be worried that you might have a urinary or bowel accident while making love. Your loved one may be too afraid he or she will hurt you if you begin sexual interactions again. Sometimes your loved one may have difficulty changing roles from being your caretaker to being your sexual partner again, and he or she may be too exhausted to even consider returning to a sexual relationship. In addition to all these issues, there are a number of areas in the brain responsible for appropriate sexual functioning that may be affected by your stroke.

If your sexual relationship was an important part of your life with your loved one before your stroke, there are many ways of overcoming these difficulties. Talking out your fears or concerns is an important first step. Keeping the communication lines open is essential in solving problems as they occur. We know that emotional distress affects our natural sexual responses, so sharing anxieties, worries, or discouraged feelings can improve our sexual interactions. Depression can affect interest in sex. Obtaining treatment for this will be important in returning to sexual interactions. The following are recommendations for improving your sexual relationship.

- Make love when you have no time pressure and you are well rested.
- Do not expect to have the perfect experience when you first return to lovemaking.
- Be patient with the process and do not let initial problems interfere with your interest in continuing your sexual relationship.
- Use relaxation techniques to make sure your body responds as naturally as possible and mental imagery which might enhance your enjoyment, such as making love on the beach.

- Try new positions that are comfortable for you, and give extra support of pillows underneath a sore shoulder or arm.
- Explore what areas of your body are sexually stimulating after a stroke, and give feedback verbally or nonverbally to your loved one about these.
- Eye contact and facial expressions are good communication techniques for those of you with speech problems.
- Do not put pressure on yourself to have intercourse if this is difficult. Being close to each other and enjoying each other's bodies is important, even if sexual intercourse is a problem. Oral-genital, or finger stimulation may be easier and more satisfying to both of you.

If intercourse is important to you and you have problems with maintaining erections, there is a "stuffing technique" where you or your partner stuff your penis into her vagina. Usually it is easier for the affected person, man or woman, to be on his/her back during intercourse and sexual activity after a stroke.

If you are dissatisfied with your ability to enjoy sex after your stroke, there are specialists you can see to improve the situation. Talk to your doctor to determine whether any of the medications you are taking may be affecting your sexual functioning. If this is true, discuss whether different medications could be tried with less negative effect. Do not stop taking your medications without a doctor's recommendation. Too many men who have stopped their blood pressure medication due to its effect on their sexual lives have ended up with another stroke shortly thereafter. Get a urological or gynecological consultation to determine what medications may be helpful to improve your sexual functioning. There are a number of penile implant surgeries that can be considered. There are also shots to enable men to maintain an erection for several hours. Discuss other devices with your urologist or gynecologist. Investigate a therapist with a specialty in sexual therapy to help you both enjoy your sexual interactions better.

Stress Management

The negative effects of stress on our lives and our health can not be underestimated. Many of you may be aware of the stress issues in your life. You may feel these have contributed to your stroke. Stress causes blood pressure and blood sugar to be higher, causes one's heart to work harder, causes problems with digestion and elimination, and causes the immune system (that fights off disease), to be disrupted.

After a stroke it is important to put your well being and your health as a priority in your life. Many men and even more women who have been parents, aunts and uncles, and grandparents have learned to put every one else's needs before their own. This leads to you not even being aware of your own needs, much less thinking of how best to take care of yourself. This lack of awareness must change. It is now important for you to put your own needs at the same level as others' needs. Defining your needs and your response to them is the first step to reducing your stress reactions.

One of your most basic needs is keeping your body healthy and well rested. Thus, you need a balance of rest, activity, and exercise. Very few of us have paid much attention to what our bodies need in our lives. We usually ignore feelings of fatigue and keep going. Listen to your body. If you are tired, take a break. Exercise is also important to keep your cardiovascular system healthy. If you are capable of it, do an activity such as walking, swimming, or pushing yourself in your wheelchair for 20 to 30 minutes three times a week. If the weather is too hot or too cold for this, go to a mall or a grocery store, or buy a stationary bike you can use indoors. Always discuss your new exercise regimen with your physical therapist and your doctor before starting an exercise program. Ensure you are considering all your medical issues, particularly if you have heart problems.

Eating healthy food is essential for your body to be at its best. Make a practice of looking at the saturated fat and sodium content of foods in the grocery store, and choose the "healthy" brand of soups, etc. Stay away from foods that are more than 20% to 25% saturated fat and are high in sodium. Reduce your beef intake and eat more fish, chicken, and turkey. Bake or broil your food instead of frying it.

Reduce your alcohol consumption to a minimum or abstain completely. Alcohol is a central nervous system depressant and therefore can make your problems from the stroke worse. Your balance, transfers, and walking may become worse: your speech may become poorer after even one drink. Drinking also puts unnecessary stress on your brain during its recovery process and may be preventing the recovery you would otherwise experience. Finally, you are putting yourself at greater risk of developing seizures when you drink. This risk is higher after a stroke anyway, and drinking alcohol can increase it further. If you were a heavy drinker before your stroke or were involved in drug use and are tempted to return to these, it is essential that you get into a program such as Alcoholics Anonymous or Narcotics Anonymous or another substance abuse program. We are now well aware that you are at more risk for stroke if you are drinking heavily or are using cocaine. Heavy alcohol use and other drug use also may impair your brain functioning in addition to what has already been affected.

Many of you have considered smoking cigarettes as a way of relaxing before your stroke. It is extremely important that you stop smoking after a stroke and develop other ways to relax. You are drastically increasing your risk of another stroke if you do not stop smoking. Research has shown that cigarette smoking causes strokes, heart disease, and many cancers. It is important for you to decrease your chances of having another stroke in every possible way .

When you are upset or depressed, try to have people you can talk to. Often it is helpful if at least one of your support persons is outside the family, since he or she will give you a different perspective on the area of concern and can be more objective than other family members. Try to set goals for solving your problems as well as for blowing off steam. Try to resolve problems with family members or friends as quickly as possible when they occur so the tensions do not build up over time. If you and your loved one are having unresolved difficulties, see if either of you can get away to another family member's or friend's house to try to have time away from each other. This can reduce some of the built up tension. Be assertive rather than passive or aggressive in your interactions with each other. State your feelings clearly and as calmly as possible without blame of the other person. "I am angry about what you just said. I felt I was being treated like a child." State how you would like to be treated. " I would like to be treated with respect."

Keep track of your mood. If you are getting depressed or anxious, try to identify what is contributing to this. Many people are more isolated socially after their stroke and need to get out of the house more frequently to improve their mood, or have friends in for a meal or visit. It is important to do activities that are fun for you. If you can not do the same things you did before the stroke, try to develop new interests or hobbies requiring less energy. Look into a stroke club or association in your neighborhood or begin one yourself. Surf the Internet for information on stroke, health, and other interests. There are chat rooms for those with specific interests. (See Chapter 10 for more discussion on the Internet).

Learn to use relaxation techniques, including muscle relaxation, focusing on your breathing, and using visual imagery. Imagine a very peaceful place where you would love to be. Visualize the place and what you can see, hear, feel, and smell. Let the tension flow out of your muscles as you breathe out. Let your breathing become smooth as you allow each part of your body to relax more and more. Focus on the parts of your body that tend to be more tense, such as your neck or your shoulder muscles, and let that tension evaporate as you breathe out. Imagine you are in an elevator at the top floor and count down as you allow the relaxation to become deeper and deeper with each floor you go down. If thoughts or worries interrupt your relaxation, focus on these and then let them flow out of your mind as you say a word to yourself such as "relax " or "peace. " If you practice these techniques, they can become a habit that enhances your ability to cope with stress forever.

Plan ahead, organize your days and weeks, and give yourself plenty of time to accomplish what you need to do. At first it is difficult to deal with the increased time it takes to get ready in the morning, and to accomplish even the most mundane things, such as taking a shower or eating a meal. As time goes on, however, this becomes easier, and you and your family can make better judgments about how long it will take to get ready for appointments or social activities. Writing down things you want to do in a day helps you to follow through more consistently and not forget important calls, tasks, or appointments.

Pain Management

Pain is a common problem after a stroke, particularly in the affected side of your body, especially in your shoulder. Usually this resolves over time as your muscles become stronger or as you realize how best to protect your joints and not to put too much pressure on them. Pillows under your shoulder and affected arm can reduce pressure on them at night. Make sure you support your elbow when sitting to prevent too much weight from pulling down on your shoulder. Back-support cushions can be helpful to prevent lower back pain if you need to sit a good part of the day.

If the thalamus of your brain has been affected, you may develop a thalamic pain syndrome. It can involve the entire side of your body weakened by the stroke. This can be more difficult to deal with and more overwhelming. If you feel your life is being controlled by your pain, it is important to find a physician and psychologist who are specialists in pain management. The physician will be able to find a medication regimen that fits your pain problems, and the psychologist will teach you pain control techniques, such as self hypnosis, relaxation techniques as described in the stress management section above, and pacing of activities to avoid out of control pain. It is important for you to be aware of the things that make your pain worse and to avoid these.

Return To Work

For many of you, return to work is foremost on your mind. This leads to a variety of questions you will ask yourself. "Will I recover well enough to handle my job? How will I handle getting around at work if I still am weak physically? Will I be able to remember what I need to and be able to think as well to handle the responsibilities I have?"

These questions can be answered in consultation with a number of professionals, as well as with your supervisor and appropriate colleagues. Your recovery from your stroke needs to be your first priority. This means you need to give yourself an adequate period of time before you consider a return to work. Going back too soon will put you into a stressful situation. This can cause you further health problems. Ask your physician how long you should take before you return to work. Even if the length of time seems too long to you, take your doctor's recommendation seriously. A vocational rehabilitation therapist can also be a tremendous help in assisting you on all work related issues.

It is usually important to return part-time initially to determine the obstacles you will have to deal with at work and not to cause yourself too much stress and exhaustion. If you have a job requiring physical strength and you have significant physical limitations, you may need to have your job supervisor determine if you could be put into a position requiring lighter duty. If your job requires a lot of thinking and analyzing, you might want to consider having a neuropsychological evaluation. This can pinpoint your areas of strength and weakness in intellectual, language, thinking, perception, learning , memory, and executive functions. With this information you can develop compensatory strategies to deal with your areas of weakness and better handle all your responsibilities when you return to work.

If it is clear that you can not return to your old job, and you are not

100% disabled, you may benefit from rehabilitation services from the State Department of Vocational Rehabilitation (DVR). They evaluate you and can support you financially for training in new areas or for returning to school or taking special course work to allow you to begin a new job. Since DVR is often flooded with applications, it is important to check back regularly with them on how your application is progressing and when you can begin your training after you and your counselor have determined your interests.

If you and your family recognize that you are no longer able to return to work, it is important for you to file a social security disability determination application as soon as possible. If your application is turned down at first, hire a lawyer who handles disability determination cases. You will not have to pay the lawyer since the government is required to pay them in disability determination cases. With a lawyer, your case is much more likely to be settled in your favor. Your social worker or case manager will be very helpful in this disability application process.

KNOWING THE SERVICES/RESOURCES IN THE COMMUNITY

Having a stroke can be overwhelming. Negotiating complex medical and social systems after a stroke makes a difficult thing even harder. It is normal to have many questions and not know which way to turn. Your treatment team will make recommendations to chart a course of recovery. The Social Worker or Case Manager in the hospital or rehabilitation program can connect you to services and agencies that can smooth your way back to the community.

Planning Your Discharge From The Hospital

It is never too early to begin thinking about your return to the community. There are many things you need to think about when you assess what you will need when returning home.

- How much assistance will I need to walk, transfer, dress, bathe, or prepare meals? Will I need help managing my finances? Your doctor, nurse, physical, occupational, and speech therapists can offer guidance or make predictions in these areas. These will depend on your progress and current level of functioning.
- If I need help, who will provide it? A family member or friend

can be trained to safely assist you. If you decide you need to hire someone to help you at home, your Social Worker or Case Manager can connect you with agencies that specialize in providing care at home. If you decide that you will not be able to return to your home, your Social Worker or Case Manager can work with you to look at options such as a Skilled Nursing Facility or an Assisted Living Facility.

- I have special care needs. Who can assist me with tube feedings, tracheotomy care, and bladder programs? A family member or friend can often be trained to provide such care at home. Your caregiver will need to practice providing your care while a nurse is available to answer questions. A home health nurse may be recommended to continue monitoring your care.
- What type of equipment will I need? Your PT and OT will recommend specific pieces of durable medical equipment you need to safely function at home. Your doctor will evaluate these recommendations and order the necessary equipment for a safe discharge.
- Is the durable medical equipment covered by insurance? Many insurance plans pay a portion of the expense. However, it must be considered to be medically necessary. If you have private insurance, the equipment may need to be approved by the insurance company before it is purchased. Unfortunately, safety equipment for the bathroom is often not covered by private insurance, Medicare, or Medicaid. You may be able to purchase these helpful supplies at a local health store or drug store.
- Who will order the durable medical equipment I need? In many hospitals and rehabilitation programs, the Social Worker or Case Manager will order and coordinate delivery of the equipment. He/ she will review potential insurance coverage for the equipment. Your approval of it should occur prior to it being ordered.
- Will I need more treatment after discharge? Your doctor and treatment team may recommend continued therapy after you leave the hospital. Home health care or outpatient services may be recommended. Your Social Worker or Case Manager can review insurance coverage for these services. He/ she may also facilitate the start of these services.

As it has been said often in this book, information is power. It is important that you have the information you need to feel in control. Request a conference with your treatment team. Ask questions. Write them down. It is easy to get lost in the agenda of the team and forget to get your questions answered. If you do not get an answer that makes sense to you, ask again. It is the job of the treatment team to educate you about stroke and your continued care needs. Please refer to the log at the end of this chapter. You can use it as a tool to document your goals, problems, and results.

Even with a great deal of planning, the transition home can be scary and frankly overwhelming. It is normal for anxiety levels to rise as discharge approaches. This is a good time to ask for extra support from the staff of professionals working with you.

Home Care Services

As discharge to home nears, you may find that the problems caused by stroke will be present in varying degrees and additional rehabilitation services are needed. Home care services of all types, ranging from health care providers to homemakers, are available in most communities. Stroke survivors frequently require home care services because of serious stroke-related problems, lack of transportation, need for intensive caregiver training, and/or distant outpatient therapy locations. It is not uncommon for survivors to have difficulty with transfer of learned skills to the home environment where numerous obstacles challenge altered functional abilities. Home rehabilitation therapists, social workers, and nurses will serve as partners as these new challenges are conquered. A distinct advantage of home treatment is applying and perfecting skills in the same place the skills will be used. Family members or friends are easily instructed and supervised as indicated by the needs of the stroke survivor.

Types of Home Care Agencies

There are multiple types of home care providers and services available today. They include home health agencies, homemaker, and home care aide agencies, private-duty agencies, independent providers and medical equipment and supply companies. Home health agencies (HHA) are generally Medicare certified and therefore subject to strict regulations set by the government. HHA's provide skilled nursing, rehabilitation therapy, medical social work, and home health aides. Homemaker and home health aide agencies provide homemakers, companions, and aides. Some of those agencies employ nurses to evaluate needs and supervise the employees. Private-duty or staffing agencies provide nurses, homemakers, companions, and home care aides. Independent providers contract directly with consumers for selected services. In this case, the consumer hires, supervises, and pays the provider. Medical equipment and supply companies provide prescribed equipment such as oxygen, mobility aids, wheelchairs and hospital beds.

Some agencies offer integrated services or so-called "one stop shopping". These agencies link with an infusion company, a home equipment company, a hospice service and/or an extended hours/private duty company. In this case, a single phone call to a central number would connect you with any of the integrated services.

Payment for Home Health Care

Medicare is the single largest payer for home health care. The following guidelines must be met in order for you to receive services under your Medicare benefit:

- the physician orders the skilled services
- the service provided must be medically reasonable and necessary for treatment of your illness or injury
- you must be homebound
- skilled nursing and/or home health services must be provided on a part-time or intermittent basis

Rehabilitation home health services are covered under Medicare A at 100% if the above criteria are met. Home health aide visits for assistance with personal care are covered as long as a skilled service (i.e., therapy or nursing) is being provided in the home. Medicare will not pay for 24-hour care, meals, prescription drugs, or homemaker services. If you are in a Medicare/HMO plan, a Case Manager authorizes home care services and visits.

Private health insurance and managed care organizations (MCO) pay for home services with pre-approval. Case managers are employed to monitor home care services and authorize the types and frequency of visits. Be a knowledgeable consumer and learn how your plan works and if you have a Case Manager!

Medicaid will cover some home care services, but it varies greatly by state. Many states are now requiring Medicaid recipients to enroll in HMOs and these numbers are expected to increase. If you have Medicaid and are in an HMO, you will have a case manager and as in any managed care plan, home care services will require preauthorization.

Consumers may pay privately for any home care services. The most frequent long-term hire is the health aide or the homemaker. Through a telephone call to any agency, you can determine the staff available for hire, qualifications of staff, and the hourly cost. Before service is initiated, the consumer should sign a fee agreement detailing costs.

Selecting a Home Health Agency (HHA)

The following questions will guide you as you make an informed decision concerning your home health services:

- How long has the HHA been in business?
- Is literature available explaining services, fees, patient's rights, and billing practices?
- How are employees selected and trained?
- How does the staff handle emergencies?
- Are references available?
- Will your health information be kept confidential?
- Will a nurse develop your plan of care and supervise the health aide?
- Is the agency Medicare certified?
- Does Joint Commission on Accreditation of Healthcare Organizations (JCAHO) accredit the agency?
- How will the agency keep in contact with your doctor?
- Does the agency employ rehabilitation therapists, social workers, dietitians, skilled nursing and home health aides or do they contract with other agencies for staff?
- Who manages employees that are contracted?
- Does the agency have only non-licensed staff, aides, companions, and homemakers?
- How does the agency handle complaints?
- Does the agency gather data and report on consumer satisfaction?
- Does the agency participate with your insurance carrier?
- Is the agency licensed?

• Can you access the agency 24 hours a day by phone?

Talk to your hospital rehabilitation team members and your family or friends about agencies that may be appropriate for you.

Assessment Tool used by Medicare Certified Home Health Agencies

Starting in July 1999, Medicare has required HHAs to collect information about your level of function at specified intervals. The new tool is the Outcome and Assessment Information Set and is known as OASIS. The nurse or therapist will complete the assessment at admission and at discharge. Medicare identifies a certification period as sixty days. That means, if you still needed skilled services beyond that time, and are homebound, then the nurse or therapist would ask your doctor to order continued treatment. You would be re-certified and have another assessment done. It is those stroke survivors with very severe deficits that require home services for the extended period of time. The majority of survivors are eager to transition to outpatient therapy, when able to leave home safely.

The assessment information will yield outcomes that Medicare will use to determine appropriate services and reimbursement for stroke home care. Quality of services will be monitored and surveyed by Medicare. The HHA will inform you of your rights in regard to answering the assessment questions. You have the right to refuse to answer questions and the HHA cannot deny services to you.

Case Management Outside the Hospital

In many communities, case management and social work services are available outside the hospital setting. The purpose of this service is to provide or connect individuals with services they need to remain in their community. The worker will assess your physical and emotional needs. In-home health services, nutritional services, transportation, and individual or family counseling can then be coordinated or provided. The worker may also help you access public benefits such as Medicaid or Food Stamps. Funding for this type of case management can come from the client or a family member requesting the service. Some agencies providing case management services are publicly funded. Therefore, their services are free or based on a sliding income scale. To find these services in your community, contact your local Office on Aging, private or public social service agency, health department social worker, hospital social worker, or case manager. Eldercare Locator 1 (800) 677-1116 is a nation-wide service that can give you information about services for the elderly in your community. There are often many services in the community that can assist you after a stroke. The key is to decide what you need and how you want the service provided.

Adult Day Care

Adult day care centers provide older adults with rehabilitation and supportive services. These centers primarily serve people who are 65 years or older. The centers are usually open Monday through Friday. There is often a daily charge. Medicaid may cover this service. Some centers provide transportation. Most centers provide a mid day meal and a snack.

Nutrition Services

There are several types of nutrition services available, depending on the recipient's ability to leave his or her home. Most communities have some form of Meals-On-Wheels. This usually consists of two meals a day, five days a week. A warm and a cold meal are delivered at the same time. There is often a weekly charge for this service. Some programs provide meals on the weekend. For elderly individuals that can leave their homes, a hot lunch is offered at many Senior Centers. In large metropolitan areas, this service may be spread among different churches, synagogues, and civic organizations. Furthermore, there are grocery stores and home health agencies that can deliver specially ordered groceries to your home. Check with your local Office on Aging to obtain details of the services in your community.

Legal Issues

After a stroke, survivors and their families may have questions related to their need for a Power of Attorney, Living Will, and Estate Planning. The National Academy of Elder Law Attorneys, the Legal Aid Bureau, and the Office of Ombudsman can connect you with an attorney who specializes in the legal issues of the elderly or disabled.

Life Line Services

An electronically linked response system is often recommended for people who live alone and are at risk for falls or other medical emergencies. These systems can be obtained through a national provider or your local hospital. Contact the Office on Aging to find out who provides this service in your community.

Income Replacement

Survivors that have not retired may wonder how they will pay their bills while they are not able to work. Many large employers offer disability insurance; a weekly check based on your regular salary. Check with your Human Resource or Personnel Department to request further information. Individuals with little or no income should contact their local Department of Social Services. You may be eligible for a small monthly check for low-income persons who are not able to work. You may want to also apply for Food Stamps and assistance with your utility bills. If you are considered to be permanently disabled, you can contact the Social Security Administration to apply for Social Security Disability Income (SSDI), Social Security Supplemental Income (SSI), or both. You may find it helpful to contact a social worker to assist you with the application process. You can also call the Social Security Administration to request assistance with the application.

Transportation

You need to talk with your doctor about your ability to drive. It is likely that you will need to rely on others for transportation, at least for a while. This is a great thing to request from those who have said, "Please let me know how I can help." Unfortunately, there are few resources in most communities for individuals who are not able to access regular transportation systems. Contact your local Department of Transportation to find out what programs are available for persons with disabilities.

Mental Health Services and Support Groups

It is very important to seek care when you are feeling emotionally overwhelmed by the changes in your life after a stroke. Many rehabilitation programs will offer counseling by psychologists or social workers. This service is often covered, at least partially, by insurance. Your local Mental Health Center can also provide counseling and support services. A Stroke Support Group can also help survivors find the emotional support they need. This is a wonderful way to find out how others have coped with the emotional and physical challenges of stroke. Refer to Appendix II for information on how to contact the American Heart Association or the National Stroke Association for a listing of Stroke Support Groups near you.

PREVENTING COMPLICATIONS AND RESTORING A FULFILLING LIFESTYLE

On returning home, it is essential that the stroke survivor follow the medical advice related to controlling high blood pressure. Obtain a blood pressure (BP) machine, learn to take your BP, record the results daily or two times a day as directed, and carry the log to the Doctor's appointment. Know your cholesterol level and goal. If diabetes is a problem, know your blood sugar goal and test your blood sugar as directed. Be compliant with the medications prescribed by your doctor. Other areas that impact your life are bladder or bowel control and sexuality. Continence is achievable and the home care nurse can help you develop a reliable program. Discuss sexuality issues and concerns with the nurse as well. Refer to the log at the end of this chapter to document your goals, problems, questions, and successes.

Every stroke survivor needs to know the warning signs of recurrent stroke, and appropriate action and lifestyle changes that need to occur to prevent another stroke. The nurse will answer questions, instruct, and supervise as needed while you are in this transition period from hospital to home. The goal is to reclaim your prior lifestyle to the fullest extent possible. The nurse on your behalf can access physicians, medical social workers, rehabilitation therapists, and dietitians. Continued medical supervision by a primary care physician is highly recommended. If a rehabilitation doctor was involved in your care following the stroke, then continue visits so that your rehabilitation progress can be monitored and complications averted. Rehabilitation physicians who specialize in stroke can be located in practice at rehabilitation hospitals, hospital rehabilitation units, or outpatient rehabilitation centers.

Home Safety and Comfort Measures

The majority of stroke survivors will return home either from the acute care hospital or the rehabilitation facility. Home is a wonderful place to be. New disabilities, may pose serious challenges. Home modification and adaptation will depend on an individual's limitations and capabilities. The PTs, OTs, and SLPs, as specialists of mobility, daily living skills, communication, and swallowing strategies, will provide expert recommendations that enhance performance and safety. Social Workers will provide information about community resources.

Ideally, these tips will start you thinking of adaptive equipment that you may find useful for your activities of daily living. For bathing, grooming, homemaking, and meal preparation aids, talk to your OT. Recommendations from your home OT will allow customization to your specific needs and capabilities. Look for self-help items in pharmacies, kitchen specialty stores, and health catalogues. Some items are very expensive, so discuss your needs with the rehabilitation staff. They can guide you in the procurement of adaptive equipment as well as referral to home modification specialists.

CONCLUSION

A stroke is probably the most challenging event you and your family will ever experience in your lives. The way you approach the challenges that you face has everything to do with the quality of life you can achieve. The love and support you can share with each other throughout the process gives each of you the strength you need to deal with the problems that may arise. Making sure that each family member has his needs met and someone to appreciate and encourage him is essential to harmony, even during the stressful situations that can arise. This is a difficult phase in your lives, but one that can bring each of you closer to each other. It can help you individually to develop internal strength that you did not know you had. It can also help you to see what the important issues are in your life and to stop getting caught up in less important details. Be patient with yourself and others as you continue on this new life journey, and attempt to add life to years.

Figure 9.1 Tips for Safety and Comfort in the Home

- Secure all floor coverings at the edges or where holes exist
- Take up any loose throw rugs
- Avoid wax on any floors
- Keep pathways free of clutter and electrical cords
- Secure stair pads and repair loose steps
- Check that handrails are tightly affixed to the wall
- Remove doors or moldings to increase width for walkers or wheelchairs
- Purchase a device that can decrease the width of the wheelchair
- Rent a hospital bed if elevated position or in bed care is needed
- Buy an incline wedge to achieve upper body elevation on a standard bed
- Add a bed board to provide a firm surface when mattress is soft or sagging
- Place blocks under the bed frame to elevate the height of the bed from the floor
- Place a 4-inch foam mattress on the mattress to elevate surface height
- Replace foam mattress once it is soft and flimsy
- Use a plastic tablecloth on top of the mattress to prevent soiling
- Keep all equipment in good repair
- Keep a phone with programmed numbers nearby when home alone
- Consider carrying a portable or cell phone as you move about the house
- Use an electronic "life line" to summon assistance
- Have a bell or baby monitor to call for help when you are apart from the family
- Have an easy to turn on light by your chair and bed
- Ask family to set up your environment before leaving you alone
- Use an insulated mug to keep water or juice available for you
- Have smoke detectors on each level and a fire extinguisher in the kitchen
- Use an old cutting board as an incline board for a reading surface
- Use anti-slip fabric from the dollar store to secure plates, pots, cushions, etc
- Set up a card table for dining when accessing the dining room is impossible
- Use a commode chair when accessing the bathroom is impossible
- Sit in an armchair with a pillow placed in the small of the back
- Use a firm cushion to elevate the seat of the armchair if needed
- Place your feet on the floor when sitting in the wheelchair
- Use a cushion in the wheelchair for comfort
- Support the affected arm on a lapboard or a trough device on the wheelchair
- Install grab-bars in the bathroom, at the toilet, bathtub, or shower
- Purchase a raised toilet seat or safety bars that surround the commode
- Use a stable bath seat for tub or shower
- Keep a logbook nearby for you or your caretaker to write down questions or messages.

Table 9.1 Making a Plan for Myself

1. What are my problems?
   The answers to the question and the problems are yours to describe. The problem you may have depends on your own particular situation and your concerns.

   1. _____
   2. _____
   3. _____

The answers to the question of goals are also yours to describe. It is helpful not only to specify what you wish to accomplish, but how much, or how fast, or how independently. When answering the question about what results you find have been achieved, it is helpful to specify not only what the results were but where or when it happened. The answers to the question about what works may also be your ideas or equipment you have found useful. It is helpful not only to specify what you do to contribute to the results, but how you go about it. "How often" or "where" or "when" are some additional questions to help make your statements more specific.

2. Following my plan

Participation: Agreement (A) Confirmed Agreement (CA) Statement (S) Specific Statement (SS)			
Date	Status/Progress	Goals	What Works
	☐	☐	☐
	☐	☐	☐
	☐	☐	☐
	☐	☐	☐

10

Technology and Stroke

MICHAEL ROSEN
JOHN NOISEUX
CHERYL TREPAGNIER
AUDREY KINSELLA
MATHEW ELROD
RICHARD KELLER
CARRIE CLAWSON
JENNIFER HENDRICKS
BRENDAN CONROY

The authors of this chapter all have something to do with technology. We suggest it to patients. We test it in the lab. We design it; write papers about it; teach therapists, engineers, and doctors about it; sometimes we even dream about it. You probably couldn't pick us out of a crowd; we usually keep our lap tops, electronic organizers, and cell phones put away. Our conversation goes beyond computers and generally touches on all the same topics that come up in your home. But despite our ordinary lives and unremarkable appearance, we do share a zeal for technology. Our enthusiasm comes from knowing just how much *things* – products that are on the market now, many of them not terribly expensive – can do to make your lives and our lives easier and fuller. These devices range from the simple and obvious (like knives and forks with big knobby grips to make them easier to hold onto when grip is weak) to the apparently miraculous (like computers you can talk to).

Nothing would make us happier than to learn that reading this chapter, and following up on the information it offers, brings you to agreeing with our point of view – especially if you started off feeling anxious or suspicious or intimidated by technology. If you have any of these feelings, you have a lot of company. At more than one professional meeting recently, in hotel conference rooms filled with people whom you might assume would be the masters of all that IBM, Sony, Microsoft, etc. have to offer, the speaker asked for a show of hands. How many people, he or she asked, still have a VCR endlessly flashing 12:00, or "Set Clock." Each time, at least a third of the audience chuckled with embarrassment and raised their hands. So you see, it's not uncommon to feel worried that some device will turn out to be too hard to use and will frustrate you instead of becoming a useful tool for accomplishment and pleasure.

But: the good news is that despite obvious examples to the contrary, useful electronic and mechanical products are being better designed these days – "better" meaning friendlier, easier to learn, more appealing – than they have ever been before. Not only that, but the products we'll talk about in this chapter include not only special assistive technology designed for people with disabilities, but also devices that can be found in Radio Shack, airline catalogs, Sears, and Sharper Image, for example. This means that the products have to be designed for use by people who don't have rehabilitation professionals nearby armed with big thick user manuals to provide instruction in their use. The products have to be easy enough for you to use them capably.

More good news: our population is getting older, needs more help in everyday activities, and their needs are being met. The growth of the baby-boom population is a topic that seems to come up in the news regularly. The boomers are in their forties and fifties, and there are a lot of them. As arthritis kicks in, low back pains act up, and vision and hearing fail, high- and low-tech products are proliferating that keep these ordinary aspects of aging from causing handicaps in the acts of everyday living. Also, those same boomers, and the generation-X and adolescent populations right behind them have more discretionary income than in times past. This means that there's a market for convenience technology, devices aimed at minimizing life's chores. Remote controls for home entertainment products are more common in the home than pencil sharpeners. And in the age of home computers, the Internet, cell phones, pagers, and car instruments to alert the driver by speaking synthetically, people in the Western or Westernized world expect technology to be all around them.

So the message for people with strokes, and their families is that there's a lot of technology out there to chose from – and more on the way. Even if a product is being marketed primarily for the convenience of people with able bodies, or to compensate for the effects of aging on those otherwise able bodies, for people who have had strokes, it could turn out to make the difference between independence and dependence. And on top of adaptable mass-market products, there is assistive technology – often abbreviated AT – developed specifically to support you and other people with disabilities. Our purpose in the rest of this chapter will be to take the mystery out of technology.

We want to demystify and organize this sprawling topic for you and put you in a position to pursue additional resources which are listed in Appendix A. We'll equip you with some terminology and with some questions to ask yourself to figure out your needs. We'll suggest kinds of professionals and support groups to help you and your family understand and decide. Think of yourself as a consumer, not as a patient. The world is a hardware store stocked with things that may be useful to you. This chapter should get grubby and dog-eared as you come back to it repeatedly to find out what's in the store, where it is, and who can give needed advice to make effective and cost-effective choices.

So what can this technology help you with? Well presumably you want the same things out of life that everyone else does, stroke or no stroke. You want to experience joy. You want to be connected to communities of people like yourself. This doesn't mean just stroke-related groups. This means interests and beliefs that distinguish you: religion, stock car racing, quilting, gourmet cooking, investing, Irish music, etc. You want independence, but not always. Doing yourself what you used to do yourself might be a goal. You want help for the rest – something or someone to take the place of lost abilities or supplement weakened abilities. And there's mobility, the freedom to be where you want to be, and maybe therapy, continuing professional input to keep your rehabilitation going as far as it can go.

And what do you need or want to do to get all you can from life? Here's a short list of life activities that you may need or want to undertake:

- Communicating (aloud or in print or electronically)
- "Mobilating" (getting around on foot or in a wheelchair)
- Driving (in a licensed road vehicle – a car or a van)

- Playing (you name it: sports, teams, social life, organizations, the outdoor life, etc.)
- Taking care of yourself (dressing, washing, etc.)
- Staying organized (keeping track of appointments, money, phone numbers, etc.)
- Using your home (managing your life at home, making use of what it offers you)
- Working (doing and keeping your job – your old one or a new one)
- Using a computer (for all things people do with computers, especially surfing the World Wide Web)

So there we have it, the outline for our chapter. In the text that follows, we'll talk about how readily available devices from the lowest low-tech to the highest high can be used in communication, mobilation, driving, playing, self-care, staying organized, home living, work and using a computer and getting on the Web. Appendix A includes a list of references and other resources you'll be able to use to pursue any of these topics further.

One last bit of generalization: You'll find in most of the sections below that four alternatives are usually available to you when you need assistance with an activity.

- Decide with your family or whomever you live with that if you can get a little help on a regular basis with setup (turning the shaver on, putting the checker board on your lap tray, etc.), you can do the activity yourself.
- There is helpful technology meant for people in general (cute phones with big buttons, jar openers for tight jar lids, remote controls for almost anything) which can pay off big for making you independent.
- There are mass-market devices available which you can use only if they're suitably modified by a trained rehabilitation engineer, an occupational therapist, a good mechanic, or carpenter, or your Aunt Sara – the industrial arts teacher.
- And, there is AT on the market aimed directly at the particular combination of skills and activities that you have in mind – technology usually well known to a rehabilitation engineer and other specialists in assistive technology.

Remember that if you're determined to do something and the technology you imagine just can not be obtained in one of these four ways, it may sometimes be possible to have a device custom designed and built for you. If you happen to live near a college with an engineering school (especially if it has a biomedical engineering department) or if the place you did your rehab has a rehabilitation engineering service with design and fabrication capability, make some contacts with these people. Cost may be an issue, although the college approach may lead to a project done by students at little or no cost. In that case, professional quality, timeliness, and accountability may be problems. The national organization of rehabilitation engineers and others who deal with AT is called RESNA, (the organization formerly known as the Rehabilitation Engineering Society of North America) See Appendix A for their phone, address, etc.

COMMUNICATION SYSTEMS AND TECHNIQUES

People who have difficulty talking, understanding, reading or writing need the advice of a speech-language pathologist (SLP). (See chapter 7). Your family members and friends can use the SLP's guidance to help make your interaction with them more successful. You yourself may benefit from speech-language therapy, especially in communication groups, which are less expensive and give you experience communicating with a variety of people.

There are also techniques, some 'low-tech' and some 'high-tech', that have been helpful to some people. Even if you can't read as you used to, you might find that you can recognize and distinguish people's names. Perhaps you can point to a name on a list to ask your spouse about what's new with an old friend, or your daughter, or grandchild.

Photos can be helpful to people who don't recognize printed names – having photos of the people important to you on the refrigerator can help you ask about them, or tell someone to contact them.

You might try a communication book – a little book with common phrases or pictures of common situations and objects. There are books made for people with language problems from stroke. There are also books made for people who are going to a foreign country whose language they don't speak. Which approach will be more helpful depends on the characteristics of your communication problems and strengths.

If you cannot tell people in words what you want and are having trouble with reading and writing, you may still make gains in these skills over time. Techniques that don't work for you now may be worth trying again in a few months, and if not then, in a couple of years. Improvement, even if it is slow, continues.

Some people who have had a stroke cannot spell correctly but can come up with the first letter of the word they want to get across. Once your family member understands the topic of the communication – for instance, that there's something you want for dinner, then you can help to get the message across by pointing to the first letter of what you want on an alphabet page in your communication book, or an alphabet page. If you're wishing for ravioli, pointing to "R" will help your family member figure that out.

Whatever technique you are using, it helps if everyone relaxes and accepts that there will be occasions when the message just doesn't manage to get across. Sometimes it is best to let it go, and try again another day.

There are computerized devices that talk, display pictures, and/or print out text on their screens and on paper. Some of this technology – sometimes called Augmentative and Assistive Communication systems, AAC for short – may help you. Costs for electronic devices range from less than $100 to several thousand dollars. Companies manufacturing these device have representatives who will gladly show you the products' features. It is very difficult, however, for a company's representative to give you unbiased advice. After all, they believe in their products, and they want to sell them. It is not advisable to invest in a communication device without guidance from a speech-language pathologist specializing in stroke. S/he knows about communication devices or will consult with someone who does.

There are also many devices and services to make the telephone easier to use for persons with varying degrees of impairment. If you have limited use of one arm, things such as headsets that fit like walkman headphones can free up your more effective arm for dialing, looking up a phone number, and taking down information. There are phone shoulder crutches that allow you to hold the phone between your head and shoulder without having to tilt your head much. You might get some help from inexpensive speaker-phones with large buttons. These are available in many chain pharmacies and discount department stores. The combination of a well-positioned speaker telephone and a mouthstick (a rod for poking keys, designed to be held in your mouth) can also allow some people to use a phone. Other phones cycle through stored phone numbers when you press a button or puff into a "puff-sip tube." A button or puff then dials the desired number. It is also important to know that there are various services that may make using a telephone easier available from many local telephone companies. Some are free. Among these are free operator-assisted dialing for those who register with the phone company, and voice dialing where you simply speak the name of the person you wish to call.

TECHNOLOGY FOR "MOBILATING"

That's not a real word – mobilating. But we needed a shorter way of saying "getting around on feet or wheels over distances and in settings where one would normally walk rather than drive". (In the rehab business, this area of expertise is known simply as "mobility".) Depending on the effects of your stroke, walking – with or without assistance – may still be in the cards. If not, than switching to wheels and being propelled by your own power, by someone else, or by electric motors will probably make sense. This section is about this need and these options.

Walking

Walking (or "ambulation" or "gait") may be partially or significantly affected after your stroke. A physical therapist is the rehabilitation professional who specializes in assisting your return to the safest and most independent level of function appropriate for you. There are three major types of equipment used to assist walking: "ambulatory assistive devices," orthotics, and "electrical stimulation." The first two are a lot more common than the third.

Walkers, crutches, and canes are the three standard types of *ambulation assistive devices*. The primary goal of these assistive devices is to help you walk with stability (keep you steady even when terrain is uneven or there are people around who might jostle you) and ensuring safety (keep you from falling and getting hurt).

- Walkers come in various flavors; they vary in height, width, and style. Some have no wheels, some have wheels on two legs, some on four. Brakes, fold-down seats, and other features make some models fancier (and heavier). Most fold flat to stow and transport easily.
- Crutches are made in the axillary style (the usual kind which come up under the armpit) or forearm style (which end at a cuff which wraps around the forearm). The most common ambulatory assistive device used by people who have had strokes is a cane. The variety of canes seems nearly infinite. There are straight wood canes, metal adjustable canes, and "quad canes" (which end in four rubber tips for extra stability). How to make these choices? Generally your physical therapist will assess and advise you on this. There's still plenty of room to express your preferences or experiment a bit without ignoring her/his advice.
- Orthoses (or orthotics; in other words braces) also help some people who have had strokes to walk with greater safety and independence. Braces in general serve to keep a joint at a desirable angle without the wearer's own muscles having to do this. Braces stiffen a joint or at least set limits on its motion. The orthoses used most often after a stroke are ankle-foot orthoses, also called AFOs. AFOs are typically used to keep your toes (on the side affected by your stroke) from dragging ("foot-drop") and more generally to give you better control of your gait. An AFO, if you need one, would be custom-made for you or ordered off the shelf if a standard size would fit you well. They're made of stiff but light-weight materials and have either rigid backs or ankle joints.

A newer and more complex type of assistive technology for assisting walking is electrical stimulation, a gentle application of electric current from a battery through stick-on electrodes. Imagine Band-Aids, not needles! Electrical stimulation can be used in two ways. It may be used to provide a tickling buzzing sensation to help you judge when you are using a muscle, in other words to tell you when you are activating it. This is one form of so-called biofeedback.

Electrical stimulation can also be used to artificially turn a muscle on at appropriate times – to make a muscle work as if you were controlling it. This is called functional electrical stimulation. For people who have had strokes, it is most commonly applied to the muscles in the front of your shin that raise the foot. It is an alternative to an orthosis for preventing foot drop. This technique was first tried in the early 60s so it's not exactly new, even though it may sound a little wild.

With all the different types of technology available to help you walk safely and independently, you'll most likely work with a physical therapist to determine which is appropriate for you and to get the necessary training.

Wheelchair Use

If you have difficulty walking because of your stroke, especially traveling longer distances on foot, there is assistive technology to help you get out and participate. From the bedroom to the living room or home to work, wheeled mobility may greatly improve the quality of your life. There are many things to consider when you are thinking about wheeled mobility options. What type of mobility aid is right for me? Where will I use it? How will I transport my chair or scooter from home to mall, for example, if I want to use it in both places? Most rehab centers can refer you to an expert in this topic or deal with it on site. Occupational therapists, physical therapists, rehabilitation engineers, and other specialists typically work as a "seating and mobility" team to evaluate your needs and abilities and make equipment recommendations.

The main types of wheeled mobility are manual wheelchairs, power wheelchairs, and motorized scooters. (The second and third of these have battery-powered electric motors.) For people with good function in one arm and/or leg, a manual chair can often meet their needs. Manual wheelchairs with seats designed closer to the ground ("hemi-height" wheelchairs) allow you to pull the chair along using your foot, in addition to using your hand on the push-rim of the wheel, if possible. For persons for whom independent mobility is not presently an option, manual chairs are also usually selected. In these cases the wheelchair is standard height and is propelled by a care giver pushing on the "pushcanes" attached to the wheelchair back. The main advantage of a manual wheelchair is its ease of transport when not in use. Most can be folded and placed on the rear seat of a car or in the trunk. Some manual chairs have quick release wheels that allow them to fit in even tighter spaces when they are stowed.

Powered mobility is particularly suited for people who have greater distances to travel or who don't have the endurance or function to use a manual wheelchair. Two types of powered mobility are available: power wheelchairs and scooters. Many people have an easier time accepting the idea of using a scooter perhaps because its appearance is less intimidating and more mainstream. Scooters are also typically less expensive. They can be easier to transport by car as they generally can be taken apart into several pieces and stowed. On the other hand, the weight of the scooter pieces can be prohibitive for loading into a car for someone who has had a stroke or for an older care provider. Another shortcoming you may encounter with a scooter is that its controls are not very adaptable. A power wheelchair lets you change to a different type of joystick, relocate it from the middle to the right side, adjust turning speed, etc. With a scooter you're pretty much stuck with handle bars in the conventional location. In addition, scooters do not come in as many sizes; they typically can't accommodate the very large or small rider and they don't allow as many options for adapted seating. This means that the seat and the back cannot be modified much to accommodate the user's shape and changes over time.

Much greater flexibility is available with power wheelchairs. Features like head support, adjustable back and seat angles, alternative controls, movable arm rests and much more are all commonplace in power wheelchairs. And this doesn't just mean during the initial purchase. A wheelchair can accommodate changes in control needs and seating systems over time to meet a user's evolving needs. Power wheelchairs do tend to be more difficult to transport. Typically you will use a wheelchair van (one that has a lower floor and includes a ramp or lift to allow entry) or accessible mass transit (e.g., buses fitted with lifts, elevator-accessible subway systems, etc.). This gets you and your chair from points A to B with you in it. Transferring out of it onto the seat of a car, for example, may make less sense since most power chairs aren't readily knocked down to be stowed. Other options include the use of an easily stowed manual wheelchair on occasions when it is not possible to transport the power chair. In these cases, your caregiver will propel the manual chair for you at your destination.

Among the issues to consider when selecting a wheeled mobility aid are the places you plan on using it. Your new mobility device needs to be able to go where you need it. You'll want to consider its weight and size to figure out if it can get into the spaces you need it to. The seating and mobility professionals you're working with may be able to help you with an evaluation of your living and working areas. Will it fit through the doors in your home? Are there narrow hallways and tight squeezes between major pieces of furniture? Are there steps to the front door? These issues should be kept in mind during the selection process. They can influence the type of device (wheelchair or scooter) and even the brand (Brand A's wheelchair fits you and gets through the doors, while Brand B's wheelchair fits you but is an inch too wide to get into the bathroom). Sometimes wheeled mobility users find that adjusting their homes to accommodate their wheelchair or scooter enhances their independence and allows them to conserve energy. Focus on the areas you'll want to use most often on the most accessible level of the home. Some modest structural changes may be needed to enhance independence and access in the home. You might need to widen a doorway or put in a ramp, for example.

Within the home, other aids to mobility may include devices that allow you to travel from one level to another if you have difficulty walking up and down stairs. A stair glide is essentially a seat on a rail that travels up and down a staircase. You sit down on the seat, put your feet on the foot rest, press a button, and you're headed up or downstairs with an electric motor doing the work. A chair glide can benefit people with strokes who can ambulate short distances but are unsteady on stairs, as well as those who use a wheelchair but can transfer safely to another seat. Typically a second, usually manual, wheelchair would be used on the other level of the home. For users unable to transfer safely, or for those who will be using a power wheelchair on more than one level of the home, a platform lift can be used to transport the user and his/her wheelchair to a different level. Like a stair glide, a platform lift travels up the staircase. Both the stair glide and a platform lift fold up to provide a clear path on the stairs for other users. It should be noted that not all staircases can accommodate these types of lifts. Many residential stairwells are too narrow to accommodate a platform lift, but stair glides can fit into narrower ones. Residential elevators are also available. They are expensive but can accommodate a wheelchair and its user.

So now you are equipped with some fundamental knowledge that should help you think through your needs with family members and the seating and mobility team at your place of rehab. This is a particularly well-developed area of technology for people with strokes and other disabilities. There is a much greater variety of wheelchairs and scooters out there now than a decade or two ago. People who use chairs and other rolling ambulation systems are also a much more common sight than ever before. This is all good news for you – more choices, and less stigma.

ADAPTED DRIVING

You've had a stroke and want to drive. Of course; it's as American as apple pie. It's a symbol of adult independence and competence. You probably remember getting your license as what set you apart from the kids some decades ago. In most places in the U.S., where public transportation is inadequate, not driving means being driven. This can feel like a step back. That this reduction in licensed mobility happens to most of us for one reason or another when we hit our seventies or eighties doesn't help much.

So what are the issues? Top of the list, of course, is can you drive and do it safely? Your state motor vehicle bureau will expect you to meet all the usual standards for holding a license. Another question is: Who can test you to find out your prospects for driving, and train you if you have a shot at it. And then there's technology. You'll probably be surprised at the number and variety of adaptations there are for drivers with disabilities. They range from simple mechanical add-ons that permit an otherwise standard car to be driven without using one's feet or with only one hand, to elaborate and expensive van modifications that permit the vehicle to be driven from a wheelchair with virtually no physical effort. A big question too is "Who pays for it?" What we'll try to do here is deal with each of these topics in brief and then point the way to sources for more information.

The hospital where you did your rehab will most likely be able to direct you to an adapted driving program. Not all rehabilitation hospitals have such programs on site so your own institution may or may not have one of its own. In fact, adapted driving specialists are not so common that you'll necessarily be able to find a program near you.

These professionals are most commonly occupational therapists or other allied health providers with special training and certification.

Once you get hooked up to an adapted driving program, you will be evaluated in a variety of ways. You'll be given various tests to assess your vision, your reaction time, your awareness of what's going on around you, your judgement, and so on. Some tests may be conducted using a simulator – like a video driving game. You may even take the wheel of a car or van in a big open parking lot with the tester sitting next to you. The outcome of all this should be a thumbs-up, a thumbs-down, or a question mark. Your driving abilities may be judged to be unimpaired, in which case you'll either go right back to driving or repeat the standard tests to renew your license. Or you may be told that, considering the amount of time that has passed since your stroke, your present abilities indicate that you're unlikely to drive again. (At that point, it would probably be a good idea to ask the physician who has been overseeing your rehab to offer a second opinion about your chances of making major gains in the abilities which underlie driving. The doctor should have access to the driving evaluator's report.) The middle ground is the determination that continued recovery, some specialized driver retraining, and effective vehicle modifications may bring you to the point where you can drive again.

In any case, the adapted driving professional evaluating you will be keeping in mind the range of special equipment that might make sense for you. If you have hemiplegia – a weakness on one side – he or she may evaluate you with what we used to call a "necking knob" back in the 50s. This makes it easy to steer with one hand. If you can use your left foot more easily than your right, the pedals can be adapted to make use of your stronger side. In other words, the question is not how well you can drive a standard car, but how well you and some vehicle modifications can "collaborate" to produce safe and effective driving.

Another player in this business is the vehicle modifier. These are essentially custom car shops which specialize in installation of adaptations for drivers with disabilities, and the modifications of the vehicle body and chassis which may be required. These changes can be substantial, especially in the case of vans to which a lowered floor, raised roof, tie-down equipment (to secure wheelchairs during travel) and a powered lift must be added – along with all the specialized driving controls – to accommodate a passenger or driver in a wheelchair. If there is more than one such shop in your region, there will generally be a bidding process in which the vehicle modifiers compete to be the lowest bidder after the agency paying for the modification posts a request for bids.

Which brings us to the money question. Each state goes about this process in a slightly different way, but most commonly it is your state's vocational rehabilitation agency that is likely to pay for driving adaptation needs if the case worker working with you judges that you are likely to return to work and need to drive in order to commute to work. This judgement is not made lightly, in particular since the cost of some of the more substantial vehicle modifications can equal or exceed the cost of the car or van itself! One common arrangement is that the driver's personal resources must cover the cost of a suitable vehicle while the agency will pay for the adaptations.

The adapted driving evaluator/instructor you work with will be able to show you pictures, catalogs, Web sites on the computer, and even actual vehicles to acquaint you with special equipment which may be appropriate for you. You may see gas and brake "pedals" that are operated by hand; steering wheels that are placed off-center and at odd angles to accommodate one-handed use and require only an ounce of force to turn; and even jet fighter-style joysticks that do steering, acceleration and braking all in one, like the usual control on a powered wheelchair. Some or none of these may be appropriate for you. The professional working with you will teach you what you need to know and will guide your decision.

If, for some reason, your rehab hospital cannot get you started on the issue of adapted driving, a call to your state vocational rehab agency is in order. An alternative is getting in touch with ADED, the Association of Driver Educators for the Disabled, or the AOTA, the American Occupational Therapy Association. See Appendix A for more details.

PLAYFUL TECHNOLOGY

Recreation, leisure, play, sports—these are the things we do by ourselves, for ourselves, and with others when we're free from the responsibilities of everyday life. A stroke doesn't change the drive to have fun, only the way we perform and involve ourselves in these activities. Technology for play ranges from high tech – such as rudder pedal adaptations on a private airplane; to low tech – such as a one-handed device for holding playing cards. (These are real examples!) Adapted recreation technology provides tools for improving one's ability to participate in leisure activities that would otherwise be difficult or impossible. Almost every sport or game has been adapted with tools or variations of play to suit someone with capabilities limited due to a stroke. Picture a checkers board with large cone-shaped checkers. And there are a variety of specialized games that were specifically designed to be played despite an impairment. How about a horseshoe-like game played with bean bags – much lighter than iron horseshoes?

A garden variety example of adapted leisure equipment for someone with a stroke would be a one-handed book holder. After all, reading is recreation. Another example is a balance aid such as a walker to make some hiking feasible. Something as simple as a wheelchair laptray may help with table-top activities. Changing the way a recreational task is traditionally done can be an effective solution as well. If a family member baits several fish hooks ahead of time, the angler with a stroke might be more independent in the fun part – catching fish and making up stories about how big they were. What makes an activity enjoyable and what steps are involved to get to the fun? You and your family can plan ahead and figure out how to help you be more nearly independent.

Many simple and inexpensive devices for recreation are available in the same catalogs that offer assistive technology in general. North Coast Medical (www.ncmedical.com), Maddak, Inc. (www.maddak.com), and Sammons Preston (www.sammonspreston.com) are three well known catalogs in the world of assistive technology offering these kinds of devices. Imagine a portable ball ramp or a ball pusher that allows bowling from a wheelchair. Many of the devices in these catalogs would typically be used in the home environment. But eating aids, for example, are just as applicable at the ball park as at home.

Ideas or resources for more specialized adaptations to equipment can be located through publications aimed specifically at people with disabilities such as the monthly magazine *Sports 'n' Spokes*, or the well known publication *Spinal Network*. These publications offer stories and information on a wide variety of topics and usually give the numbers and addresses of relevant associations and equipment vendors.

There are also state and university programs with information and newsletters that are good resources. The Delaware Assistive Technology Initiative (DATI) is an example of a State program with a newsletter offering updates, information, publications, and even a section for people selling used AT equipment. Purdue University and the USDA AgrAbility Program have a newsletter called *Breaking New Ground* designed for more rural users of AT for "cultivating independence for farmers and ranchers with disabilities." The Program has expanded beyond Indiana to include Colorado, Delaware, Texas, and Utah. These newsletters are usually good places to see pictures of and read about specific custom modifications to devices and equipment now used for purposes including recreation. And, of course, there is all kinds of information available on the Internet about associations, manufacturers, equipment, and personal experiences regarding the area of sports, recreation, and play. There is a section later in this chapter about how to use a computer to get on the Web; and the resources listed in Appendix A include some specific Web sites.

A little philosophy: technology used for play should meet your goals. So ask yourself what your needs really are. If the adaptations needed to achieve exactly the same level of involvement in the same activities you enjoyed before a stroke are too costly, are technically too difficult, or create a whole new set of problems, you might want to rethink your goals. The flatter, smoother trail might let you enjoy the air and the friendship as much as the tough one. Can you indulge you competitiveness as readily with "knock hockey" (one-handed) as with a real slap shot on ice? Try and see.

TOOLS THAT HELP YOU TAKE CARE OF YOURSELF

Many self-care activities such as dressing, bathing, grooming, and eating can be made easier with the use of low-tech aids, as discussed in Chapter 8. You may already be familiar with some of them, like reachers, tub seats, bedside commodes, and adapted eating utensils. If you haven't needed or come across this handy hardware, but you or your family believe you may benefit from it now, ask your occupational therapist or check out some of the catalogs listed at the end of this chapter.

Dressing aids are all low tech items and have been discussed in Chapter 8. Typically folks who have difficulty manipulating small objects can benefit from devices that help do up buttons and zippers. Sock aids can help individuals who have difficulty donning socks and stockings; elastic shoe laces can eliminate the difficulty of tying shoes one-handed. These types of items can be found in catalogs such as Sammons Preston (see reference section at end of chapter). An occupational therapist can help you in determining what dressing aids and techniques will be helpful to you.

There are many products that may increase your independence and efficiency while bathing. Among these are no-tech items such as washing mitts and long handled sponges. Various tub seats and benches may also be appropriate. Typically an occupational therapist can help you identify a good choice to meet your needs. Items such as hand held showers, grab bars, and push button dispensers for soap, shampoo, and conditioner are somewhat more complex in that they need to be installed. Some models of hand held showers allow you to adjust the height of the showerhead (that is – they let the showerhead slide up and down vertically on a tube). This is beneficial for one-handed bathers using a shower chair or tub bench. It allows you to target the spray and place the showerhead at a comfortable height. Grab bars, (not towel racks which aren't designed to support the weight of a person and could give way unexpectedly) can also enhance your safety in the bathroom area. Whether it be transferring to a toilet or providing something secure to hold on to while stepping out of the shower, a grab bar can be very helpful. A soap dispenser mounted on the shower wall within easy reach can save you the trouble of trying to pop open bottles of shampoo (especially tricky one-handed) and may increase your safety in the shower (no lose bottles or bars of soap to trip on). Don't forget basic items like non-skid tub mats and floor mats for safety entering and exiting the tub!

An electric razor is a much safer alternative to razor blades for shaving. When buying an electric shaver, try it out in the store to make sure you are able to turn the razor on and off easily, especially if you are using primarily one hand. (Or, decide with the people who live with you that somebody will turn it on and off for you. Or look into getting somebody to make you a switch adaptation so you can do it yourself.) Also make certain you can operate the recharging mechanism or plug in the razor. A larger, lighted mirror can be helpful for shaving. This holds true as well for applying makeup, especially if you're seated and unable to use the standard-height vanity mirror.

An electric toothbrush can be easier to use when a person must use the "other," or non-dominant hand to brush. There are currently several different powered products available to assist in cleaning between teeth. These devices require good coordination and endurance of the arm, as well as good attention and problem-solving skills, for efficient and safe use. Again, make sure you are able to turn the toothbrush on and off as well as manipulate it before you purchase it (this is a good rule of thumb for all your small household appliances). Discuss this issue with your occupational therapist or physician if it is a concern, and then talk to your dentist for a specific product recommendation.

Some high-tech aids for feeding have been developed but are surprisingly expensive and not really appropriate for most people who have had strokes. Typical accommodations that may benefit you include various adapted silverware (large handles, etc), and non-skid mats for bowls and dishes to prevent sliding while you're eating. Bowls and plates with "sides," or high edges can make it easier for a one-handed eater to get some foods onto a spoon or fork (i.e. push the food onto the spoon by cornering it against the sides of the bowl or dish). For food preparation you may benefit from items such as a pot-handle holder (holds the pot handle while you stir so the pot doesn't move around), electric knives (be aware that use of a knife may not be appropriate for persons with spatial/perceptual difficulties), electric can openers, small hand-held mixers, kitchen timers, food processors, and microwave ovens. Remember also that the selection of food items can also contribute to independence in feeding and food preparation (e.g., pre-peeled baby carrots, bowtie pasta vs. spaghetti, bagged salad mixes, etc.) See the references in Appendix A for sources for some of the devices mentioned.

GETTING ORGANIZED, STAYING ORGANIZED

So many things to do! So many phone numbers to remember! Thank goodness for one of the most important technologies ever invented – the pencil! A small purse- or pocket-sized calendar, the type that lets you see the whole week on two pages, is helpful for many people. If there is a section in the back for telephone numbers in alphabetical order, so much the better. This can be very helpful for appointments, for things you must get done, and for avoiding doing things too often. Checking things off once you've done them might mean not finding yourself changing the linen twice in the same week.

Maybe you need some help with keeping track of daily tasks, like remembering when to take medication. You want to be sure not to miss a dose, and, just as important, you don't want to take a double dose. Pill containers, with compartments labeled by day or by time of day, can be bought in the drug store and may be all the help you need. Once the compartment marked "morning" is empty, you know not to take any more pills that morning. That can be much easier than getting pills out of bottles, and then trying to remember five minutes later whether you took them or not. It is easy to forget things like that, for people who are recovering from stroke, and even for people who haven't had a stroke.

You may find that calendars, notebooks and date-labeled containers are not enough to keep you from forgetting to take your pills. In that case, you may need a consistent reminder. For some people, an audible alarm watch that beeps at pre-set times will do the trick. Others may need a more specific reminder, like an organizer (a Palm Pilot, for example) on which messages can be recorded. Instead of just a beep, the reminder message will be displayed on a little screen, or even spoken out loud.

Another type of organizing support is the "spoken list." If you have trouble with reading, or with speaking or both, you might find it helpful to obtain a little computerized device that records someone's voice. For example, if you want to remember to buy a newspaper and a quart of milk at the store, your family member can speak those words into the device. Then when you get to the store, you press the button and you and the sales clerk can hear what you need.

People with stroke aren't the only ones who can benefit from supports for getting organized. From written lists to computerized calendars, a lot of people depend on these things. That's good, because it means that companies will make and advertise these helpful tools and that makes it easier for you to find them. There are catalogs, special stores, and many general-purpose stores with departments in which you can find things from "low-tech" pocket calendars to electronic devices and software programs for your home computer. For example, office-supply stores have a large selection of pocket calendars; often bookstores have them, especially around New Years and the beginning of the school year. And your local pharmacy, supermarket, and all-purpose discount stores should have a selection, too.

People with strokes affecting different parts of the brain can't all benefit from the same tools. The nice thing about 'low-tech' compartmentalized pill containers and pocket calendars is that you can try them without spending a lot of money. For more expensive items like electronic organizers and reminder devices, office supply "super-stores" may let you try them right in the store. Software programs can often be tried out in advance too. More about that in the section on making use of computers. The resource list in Appendix A will help you locate supports for getting organized.

TECHNOLOGY FOR LIVING BETTER AT HOME

People who have had a stroke are usually concerned about managing day-to-day activities and how much they'll be able to do for themselves at home. Living after a stroke means changing your routines – relearning old skills or learning effective new behaviors and techniques to accomplish and enjoy cooking, eating, exercise, taking medications regularly, monitoring your recovery and health, and controlling appliances and devices in your home.

Easy-to-use technologies that can assist in daily home routines have become readily available. Consider an appealing and fundamental example: preparing and eating good meals. There is now easy-to-use software for a home computer that provides nutritional counseling and help with menu planning. The software contains a great deal of information about the calorie and cholesterol levels of various foods and can be programmed with specific dietary instructions and restrictions that apply to you. It will help you choose the right kinds and quantities of foods and can also print out menus and shopping lists. This digital assistant can provide vital help because controlling your weight and cholesterol levels can be even more critical to your health than for people who haven't had strokes. Here are two sample products:

- Dine Healthy for Windows (Dine Systems, Amherst, NY): 800-688-1918, http://www.dinesystems.com
- Menu Mizer (Menu Systems, Ruffs Dale, PA): 800-559-3340

In addition, for a more personal approach, the American Dietetic Association offers a free service. Call 800-366-1655 to get answers to your questions from a registered dietitian.

Other enabling technologies can help you to take care of yourself at home – helping, for example, with exercise and medication by providing education and reminders. Probably the best way of looking at some of these new tools—such as automated weight scales that talk back and telephone reminder systems that instruct you on the time of day to take a pill and whether or not it's supposed to be taken with food—are a means to help you to "know what to do." We all are told things that we forget, stroke or no. These tools can help to remind you and your caregivers which items are important to track and which routines must be followed regularly.

Does that mean that machines will become annoying and not particularly wanted housemates? Not at all. Take, for example, an automated telephone medication reminder system that can easily be programmed to remind you of your daily routines. The programming can be done to speak in the voice of someone you know, such as one of your adult children or a friend. When it's time to take a pill, the telephone will be programmed to ring and the voice you know can say: "It's 2:00 P.M., Mom. Please remember to take two of your pills. The orange bottle. I love you." It's computer-generated but kind of personal. Most well-stocked drugstores also have "home health technology" sections that will let your care givers electronically monitor your blood pressure and weight.

Earlier we said that living after a stroke means changing your routines and learning effective new behaviors and techniques. If you now find things like operating a television remote control, opening drapes, and turning on a light difficult, there is technology available to make it easier. It may mean that instead of turning the knob on a lamp to switch on the light, you plug in a device between the socket and the lamp plug that allows you to turn on the lamp by just touching the lamp – anywhere on the lamp. Another technology called *X10*, available from stores such as Radio Shack, will allow you to turn on lights, fans, and other electrical appliances with a remote control. You can even purchase a "Super Remote" to allow you to operate your television, VCR, lights and fans all from one controller. This is particularly helpful for someone with a mobility impairment who can still press buttons on a remote control.

Other higher-tech devices called environmental control units or ECUs will allow you to operate the controls on a hospital bed, use a telephone, open a door, as well as operate a television, VCR, lights, and fans – all using a switch selected to be easy for you to access and operate. This switch can be a single big button, a straw that you sip on, a lever that you bump with your head, etc. Environmental control units are relatively expensive and require good memory and attention skills. It is important that someone familiar with the technology and the types of difficulties you may be experiencing assist you in selecting an ECU. Persons such as occupational therapists and rehabilitation engineers familiar with assistive technology can help determine what equipment would be a good fit to you.

Please read the section below on using the Internet where you can take advantage of organized opportunities to chat with other people who have had strokes. Also have a look at the long list at the end of Appendix C for other handy strategies and devices that can customize your home for your needs and preferences. And there's the list of sources for additional information in Appendix A to help you to know what to do as you learn to enjoy your home again after a stroke.

MAKING YOUR WORKPLACE WORK

Because the tasks people need to perform every day at work are almost infinitely diverse, the list of "technology" available to "accommodate" jobs is much too long for a chapter, much less a whole book. Anything from an electric stapler – to make stapling a one-handed task – to a screwdriver with a magnetic tip to hold the screw on may be helpful. And when it comes to figuring out who to ask for help, there are also many who can help. Occupational therapists, rehabilitation engineers, clever technicians, machinists, carpenters, and others who make things for a living; vocational counselors who may have seen similar problems; physical therapists who understand the limits of your strength and motion – all these folks may need to be involved in adjusting the tools and setting of your work. But don't forget that *you* may have the most insight into causes of difficulty. This is the vital first step in figuring out the accommodations and technology to make your work place serve you best.

It can be a frustrating trial-and-error process, but the plain truth is that some tasks that were not difficult before a stroke may need to be done in new ways. Whether it's a memory aid to keep you organized, or holders to allow you to perform a two-handed task with one hand, many devices can support your mind and your body in the work environment. Much of what's useful on the job will be mass-market devices which turn out to have particular value for people with disabilities. Custom changes to your work environment may take a little more thinking, but they can often be made from common inexpensive materials.

When considering how a person with a stroke will use technology to continue to be productive, it is important to think about how s/he will be positioned for job tasks. Before someone can work at a computer, for example, s/he must be well supported. The seat, whether a wheelchair or office chair, needs to provide comfortable, stable support in order for the individual to concentrate on the task at hand. If the chair challenges instead of assists your muscles in keeping you in a healthy advantageous position to work, your energy and attention will be diverted to trying to remain upright and reach your job materials. A person with good function in one arm needs to have that arm available to hold a tool, type, solder, paint, handle papers, turn pages in a book, etc. Good support in the chair will minimize or eliminate the use of this arm for repositioning and propping oneself up. A seating clinic, physical therapist, and/or occupational therapist can help determine the seating and positioning needs for people going back to work after a stroke.

As we pointed out above, job accommodation devices are almost limitless. They do fall into certain categories, however. Some allow you to perform tasks one-handed, such as computer use. The BAT personal keyboard (from Infogrip, Inc., at www.infogrip.com), for example, offers all the functions of an extended keyboard for one-handed use. Others are labor-saving in permitting you to do your job while applying less force or expending less energy. These include simple add-on handle extensions to give you more leverage in operating a tool or machine and devices which supplement or replace your effort by motorizing or automating a task – for example power screw drivers, voice-activated phones, or electric door-openers. Take a walk through a good office supply or hardware store or let your fingers do the walking through a catalog of standard or adapted work devices. Notice the electric scissors, electric hole punches, and electric staplers. Pay attention to the very low-tech materials like dysum, a non-skid material that keeps objects from sliding on a table; and the fancier items like computer keyboards that are set up for one handed users.

Here are some places to look for help with job accommodation (along with the Job Accomodation Network and other information sources in Appendix A):

- Your state Vocational Rehabilitation agency.
- Therapists – typically Occupational Therapists – specializing in worksite accommodation.
- Rehabilitation engineers – contact RESNA for a "Certified Assistive Technology Practitioner" in your area (www.resna.org or call 703-524-6686).

USING A COMPUTER AND GETTING ON THE WORLD WIDE WEB

Computers are everywhere nowadays. This can be intimidating for people with limited or no experience with them. It is important to remember that a computer is a tool – a very versatile one which can be a calculator, typewriter, calendar, drawing machine, music player, phone dialer, checkbook keeper, etc. etc. – but still just a tool. Like a socket wrench or a food processor, a computer is only useful if you have the parts you need. In the world of computers, the carrot slicer, meat grinder, and egg chopper components are the monitor (video screen), the CPU (the box with the electronics in it), and the software (the programs which make the computer do "intelligent" functions. Different tasks need different software. For instance, if you want to use the Internet, you will need both the software and an Internet service provider (such as America Online (AOL) that hooks you up to the rest of the world). Often people who haven't used a computer before wonder what they might use one for. Typical uses for a computer include writing (using a word processor), keeping track of finances (spreadsheets, accounting software, checkbook programs), storing information (addresses, phone numbers, recipes and appointments), and communication (using email, "chat rooms," etc. to keep in touch with family, friends, and special-interest communities such as other people with strokes). All of these tasks can enrich your personal life, but they can also make it easier to complete work tasks as well. It is important to recognize that using a computer depends on some cognitive skills such as attention, memory, organization, and problem solving. All of these could be affected by a stroke, and this can impact using a computer independently. If computer use would make sense for you but some functional problems stand in your way you can work with an OT and a rehab engineer.

Being able to keep track of expenses and balance a checkbook can be important for confidence, security, and independence. Many large banks and even investment companies now allow customers to review their finances and investments, shift funds, and pay bills by using a computer to access their Internet sites. Software such as Quicken can allow you to pay bills and set up automated monthly payments (such as mortgages and car payments) by using their software. Many busy people find these services valuable. People with strokes who may have impairments of mobility and dexterity, or limited endurance (and want to spend their energy someplace other than waiting on a line in the bank!) can find these services especially attractive.

Mobility limitations can reduce the amount of interaction you have with family and friends. One way of expanding your interaction with them and others can be by using new forms of communication. Email allows you many of the benefits of letter writing – you have the luxury of taking your time in composing and writing your thoughts. But since it is delivered nearly instantly, you and others can carry on a steady dialogue, "messaging" back and forth several times in a day. In addition, instant transmission of messages to and from "chat rooms" (virtual lounges with many people all "logged on" at the same time) allows you, via the Internet, to converse electronically with others. Support groups for many types of disabilities have web pages and discussion groups where people can share their experiences and benefit from the knowledge of others. Locating these sites is not difficult; stroke-specific sites such as National Stroke Association (at www.stroke.org) have easy links to these resources.

People with strokes interested in using computers may have concerns about how or if they'll be able to use a keyboard, a mouse, or a trackball, and perhaps how well they'll be able to see what's on the monitor. Many people who have had strokes yet have good use of one hand can learn to type proficiently with that hand. Software tutorials and books have been designed to help people relearn typing with one hand. See, for example, the TASH International catalog (that can be ordered from their site at: www2.tashint.com) for one-hand typing tutor software. Books on life using one hand after stroke (such as *How to Conquer the World with One Hand—and an Attitude*) are available through www.Amazon.com, as noted in Appendix A.

For folks with some visual impairments, larger monitors with high contrast settings can be helpful. Placement of reference materials toward the user's non-affected side can reduce reaching, muscle strain and poor posture, as well as increase work speed. Use of copy holders and book holders may also help. These items can be typically be found in large office supply stores, or through catalogs.

There are many other computer adaptations made for persons with strokes who have difficulty with the standard mouse, touchpad, keyboard, and monitor. There are reduced size keyboards for persons who can type with only one finger (for example the TASH International WinMinni), trackballs, and even minitrackballs. Some of these items can be tried at your local computer store, while others are specialty items that can be ordered from AT catalogs (for example, Infogrip, which can be reached through their web site, www.infogrip.com), or purchased from vendors.

Software is also available, some already built into the computer, that can make using the computer easier for people with disabilities. Features available for both Macintosh and Windows allow one-handed typists to perform functions that normally need multiple keys held down simultaneously. If you have difficulty getting your finger off a key fast enough to keep from getting multiple keystrokes (bbbbbbb), you can slow down or turn off the "repeat-key" feature to completely prevent this. Software to increase the size of icons and letters on the screen is also available, as is software that can read aloud documents on the computer.

Some specialty equipment and software is quite expensive, so you'll want to be sure it meets your needs. For this purpose, even if you are an accomplished computer user, it's best to consult an occupational therapist and rehabilitation engineer who can help match products to your needs.

WHO WILL PAY FOR ALL THIS?

The short answer to this question is, unfortunately: it depends. It depends on your age, the state you live in, and what private, state, or federal sources of funding you are relying on to cover the costs of your rehabilitation. The more useful short answer is that you can find out about coverage for the assistive technology you need by talking to the social worker or case manager at your rehab hospital. It's part of her/his job to know and to teach you. He should also know whether and how to look for coverage for technology while you're an inpatient and when you're an outpatient. To complement what s/he tells you, here are some general rules.

If you are covered by Medicare (you're over 65 and you've "paid in" to the system over the years), then certain pieces of standard or "tradi tional" equipment will be covered. Wheelchairs, commodes, canes, walkers and orthotics (braces) are on this short list. All of these covered items are examples of so-called *durable medical equipment*. Other traditional low-tech occupational therapy equipment, such as reachers and long-handled sponges, is sometimes covered by Medicare. This is very much a matter of entrenched policy, tradition, and "cost-containment" (that means setting a limit on how much is spent, in plain English). Don't expect it to make too much sense. For example, a commode (portable toilet) will often be paid for while raised seats for standard toilets are not.

If you are covered by Medicaid, the answer to the Who-will-pay question varies from state to state. With regard to private insurance and managed care plans, coverage for technology also varies widely. You'll need to inquire. At least partial coverage for the list of things above is fairly common among private payers. A general observation seems to be that Medicare sets the tone, and other insurance and plans tend to mirror its policies.

What about electronic communication devices, remote controls to operate appliances around the house, electronic organizers, voice re-corders, etc. – in other words all the less-traditional technology we've included in the coverage of this chapter? The news here is not great. In general these things are not covered because the various public and private sources of health insurance continue to be governed by the notion of "medical necessity." They cover what is medically neces-sary and this is often defined in a pretty narrow way. One might argue that a communication aid is medically necessary since it makes it pos-sible for an individual with a stroke to make medical needs known and thereby maintain her/his health. Or that an inability to communicate reliably can cause depression leading to failure to exercise, eat right, take medication and other behaviors which are essential to health. While sensible, such logic often makes no difference when it comes to funding for technology.

The bright side may be that since the health care reimbursement system in the U.S. is in a state of flux and is being examined and re-examined by all parties, the possibility of change is real. Some advocates for people with strokes and other disabilities have been pushing for many years for coverage of technology based on functional need rather than medical need. If this were a book on health economics, we could probably do dollars-and-cents analysis to show that public and private funds invested in helping people function independently and effectively could save our society large amounts of money, money which is now being spent supporting people who are dependent. In any case, keep an eye on the newspaper for the latest on this topic, and ask your case manager or social worker for interpretation of what you read.

When it's clear that some needed system or device will not be bought for you, it may be time to turn to civic organizations in your neighborhood. Kiwanis, Rotary Club, Knights of Columbus, the Lions, or the Elks among them, often take up worthy causes which might include raising funds for the environmental control system or computer adaptation that you need. This may be worth a try. There are also "funds in memory of _" that have a particular focus on stroke, or medical or rehab needs. You can talk to other families of stroke patients, talk to your case manager or social worker, or get on the Web and start looking around. Use searches with "stroke" or "disability" and "funding" or "support" as the topic. Also, the next section covers very briefly the law regarding an employer's responsibility to modify the workplace to meet the needs of a worker or applicant with a disability. If this applies to you, read on.

THE AMERICANS WITH DISABILITIES ACT (ADA)

This legislation, passed by Congress in 1990, is a civil rights act for people with disabilities (including the effects of stroke). It forbids discrimination in all settings. Up to that point, it had only been illegal in institutions receiving federal funding (such as schools with government grants). The ADA has five sections or "Titles" as they're known. Title 1 concerns people with disabilities in the work place. It specifically prohibits discrimination based on disability by an employer against current employees who become disabled. It also prohibits discrimination in the application and hiring process. An employer is required to provide "reasonable accommodation." This is defined as any modification or adjustment to a job or the work environment to enable an otherwise qualified applicant or employee to participate in the application process or to perform essential job functions without causing undue hardship for the employer. This means, among other things, that an employer is required to accommodate, where possible, use of wheelchairs (e.g., rearrange furniture, raise a desk, modify bathrooms, etc), and use of other assistive technology (e.g., phone head sets, reduced-size keyboards, customized setting for a computer interface, etc.). The legal definition of "Undue hardship" takes into account the size and resources of the company in determining the upper limits of expense and complexity constituting a reasonable accommodation.

Titles 2 and 3 of the ADA deal with public and private accommodation. With respect to assistive technology and people who have survived a stroke, the most important aspects of these sections of the law are their impact on new construction and on mass transit systems. The ADA specifies that public facilities and programs must be accessible. This has manifested itself in proliferation of ramps and curb cuts, new public buses with wheelchair lifts, subway construction including elevators, and trains with wheelchair spaces. In addition, the ADA mandates that businesses providing services to the public must provide reasonable accommodation where it does not cause undue hardship. Also, it specifies guidelines for architectural accessibility for new construction (e.g., wheelchair accessibility in hotels, movie theatres, shopping malls, and other public places).

The overall effect of the ADA has been to increase greatly the opportunities available for people with strokes to continue to enjoy the benefits of, and contribute to, their community and to society in general. Unfortunately, another effect has been lots of new work for lawyers dealing with suits resulting from employers' decisions to fight rather than accommodate. If you are headed back to work, there's a reasonable chance that a current or potential employer who finds you qualified will be willing to make adjustments if the cost doesn't turn out to be too frightening. Getting some advice from the Job Accommodation Network (see Appendix A) and generally doing your homework before making a pitch to an employer would be a good idea.

11

Consumers Speak Out

The Hall's Story
Pat Hall and Paul Rao

Edward Hall and his wife Pat had lived with "more happiness than most people have in a lifetime. No one could deserve a better husband. No one could deserve a better father," says Pat who then gives her husband an admiring look. Then on March 22,1988, Edward James Hall, nicknamed Bill by his grandfather, suffered a stroke. The bleeding into the left side of his brain rendered him unable to move, to communicate, or even to recognize loved ones. Bill's stroke was one of 500,000 that occurred in 1988 with 150,300 of those people dying. Stroke is the third leading cause of death and disability in America, after "diseases of the heart" and cancer. Stroke is a form of cardiovascular disease that affects the arteries of the central nervous system. It occurs when a blood vessel bringing oxygen and nutrients to the brain bursts or is clogged by a blood clot or some other particle. Because of this rupture or blockage, part of the brain does not receive the flow of blood that it needs. As a result, it starts to die. A large number of persons with stroke are survivors! Currently over 3 million Americans are stroke survivors. But stroke is a major cause of disability. Like Bill, many of these survivors are left with mental and physical disabilities and receive expensive, time-consuming and intensive, rehabilitation to try to increase their independence. Most stroke patients can benefit from rehabilitation, and today the outlook for persons with stroke is more hopeful than ever before. Because of advances in treatment and rehabilitation, many patients are being restored to a useful life.

"I remember Easter Sunday. Bill didn't even recognize our grandchildren," Pat says. "There were some tough times." The tough times included a time nine months after the stroke when Bill slipped into a deep depression once he was more aware of his disabilities. "Bill was a

235

hunter and he tried to get upstairs where he kept his guns. He indicated that he wanted to take his life," Pat said.

On May 9, 1988, Bill was transferred to the National Rehabilitation
Hospital to begin physical, occupational, and speech therapy. The
damage to his brain left him with a paralyzed right side and problems
with his speech and language, known as apraxia of speech and aphasia. "The inability to communicate is much worse than the physical
disability," Pat declares. "It locks you inside your own body- what you
think, what you feel, what you want—it's terrible."

At NRH, Bill's initial team meeting revealed an extremely supportive, intuitive, and involved spouse who was prepared to become a
co-therapist. Although Bill had a severe communication impairment
and a significant right-sided paralysis that limited walking and completion of his own daily living activities, the team agreed with Bill to
involve his spouse in all aspects of his treatment. The spouse became
the common thread connecting all three therapies. She carried over
each team goal to each therapy session and practiced each of the day's
activities with Bill in the evenings and on weekends. The patient and
spouse were encouraged at the outset to list his problems and goals
indicating what it is that together he could do, could not do and didn't
much miss, and finally what activities he could not do after his stroke
but really would like to do again. In short, the team agreed to treat the
"activity/skill area" that the patient and spouse elected.

Bill was indeed fortunate to have strong support from Pat, his family, friends, and church during his road to recovery. "They (medical
staff) tell you that most stroke patients recover as much as they ever
will within the first 6 months to a year after the stroke," Pat notes.
"But Bill recovered more *after* one year. Their [stroke patients'] tolerance is low. They tire very easily, and they can only work for very short
periods of time. But don't stop working with them," she pleads.

Pat recalled a situation in Bill's therapy. A decision was made that
he could not use a leg brace for his right leg. This brace would enable
him to walk. "I saw what he was doing at home. I had to beg. I thought
he could do more, So we tried the brace and he started to walk. It just
boosted his morale," Pat said with pride. "What he had the ability to
do doesn't always show up in the tests."

According to Dr. Paul Rao, Bill's treating SLP at the time, Pat was
an excellent advocate for her husband. Dr. Rao commented, " Pat saw
and knew more about Bill and his ability than I. She's with him every-

day. I only saw him for one hour of that day. I saw Bill progress in three ways:

- First, was his willingness to take the initiative. He would stop people in the hall and engage in communication.
- Second, was his self-awareness. He was more aware of what he could and could not do.
- Third, were his functional gains. He was willing to try different ways to communicate. If he could not say it, he would draw it. If he couldn't draw it, he would try to gesture it. If these alternative methods didn't work. . .he'd get Pat to communicate! Bill and Pat can not *not* communicate!"

After treatment was concluded, the patient and spouse had reached all of their "rehab and quality of life goals." As a result of the aggressive team approach with spouse as co-therapist, the rehab outcome was favorable. The patient achieved the selected goals permitting him and his spouse to enjoy a quality of life after stroke. It empowered them to do for each other what they both knew they were capable of as a team. They were indeed able to "add life to years" by becoming actively involved in making life skill— choices.

Following the conclusion of formal therapy, Bill and Pat joined the NRH Come Back Club (Stroke Club) because, according to Pat, "it was encouraging to talk to people who have been through the same thing. You encourage each other. There is no way to describe what it [stroke] does to our lives. With the club, you can ask 'Did you ever have such and such happen?' You know you are not the only one going through it." Bill and Pat found inspiration from stroke club members like Dick W. who gave Bill two books on "assisted fishing" to help him get back to fishing: *Products to Assist the Disabled Sportsman* by J.L. Pachner Limited and Don Kreb's *Access To Recreation*.

They also met Colonel Bill and his wife, Lydia. "The colonel was in the service and so was Bill, so they had that link. It's something to communicate about," said Pat. They added Helen and Bill B. To their list of friends. " Helen has since passed away, but I used to admire them so much. Helen could write and my Bill could talk. That's how they communicated. Bill B. and I would try to help them if they had trouble communicating together, but then Dr. Rao would threaten to put tape over our mouths," exclaimed Pat. "Bill did get his driver's license again. It was the same day as the stroke club meeting. On the eye exam part, they allowed him to write the letters down, since he couldn't say them. On the driving part, he was only marked for not signaling for a turn. We went to the Come Back Club meeting and Bill stood up, showed his license and said 'I can drive.' Then he introduced me. It was such a boost," Pat boasted. Their car is equipped with a knob on the steering wheel and the foot pedals are all on the left side. Bill and Pat have come a very long way...together...since that day in March of 1988. "You search your soul for why its happening, but there's no reason for it, " Pat explains. "Make the best of it. Time makes it better. There is a life after stroke."

Life Outside Academe
John D. Phillips

Editor's Note: Until three years ago, John D. Phillips (Phi Beta Kappa, Williams College, 1959) was a typical, successful, hard-driving Phi Bete. After earning a Ph.D. in American history from Stanford University in 1965, he was an assistant professor and vice president at Lewis and Clark College in his hometown of Portland, Oregon. The pace picked up when be left academe for a five-year tour at the U.S. Office of Education. He served as deputy commissioner for higher education in the Ford administration. The pace quickened further when he became the founding president of the National Association of Independent Colleges and Universities. The pace became frantic when he ran an executive search practice specializing in recruiting college presidents. In 1995 he had a stroke that almost took his life. This is the story of the stages he went through and the lessons he learned in his quest for optimum recovery and rehabilitation.

On Saturday, October 21, 1995, 1 did what came naturally to a 57-year-old workaholic. I finished working a brutal six-day week, and thought nothing of it. As a matter of fact, I thought I was enjoying it. I didn't notice my slurring speech as the day wore on.

An unavoidable pile-up of client, committee, and board meetings meant that I had been all over the country that week. Four round-trips— by train, plane, and rental car had— taken me to Philadelphia, New England, and California. When I returned home that

Saturday, I enjoyed a big pasta dinner with my son Jack and some of his friends in town for the Marine Corps marathon starting early Sunday morning. I was supposed to drive him to the start of the race and to be available with water at the halfway mark . I never made it to the race, and neither did my son.

I was in the kitchen of our McLean, Virginia home. I was fixing Sunday morning breakfast with my wife, Paula, and all but one of my family members. Then the stroke hit. Suddenly I sensed numbness in my right arm and quickly found I could not move the arm at all. As I tried to explain what was happening, Paula noticed I had saliva running from the right side of my mouth. She got me to a kitchen chair and had Jack hold me there while she ran upstairs to waken our daughter Jenna (a medical social worker) and daughter Katy's husband, Fred (M.D., internal medicine). In the 20 seconds or so it took for Paula to describe my symptoms, Jenna was already calling for an ambulance.

The Fairfax County ambulance crew got there in just under six minutes. The oxygen tank they brought with them saved me from far more severe effects on my brain before I reached the hospital 20 minutes later. I'm told that it was amazing what they did for me, but I couldn't even hear the siren.

Phase One

It turns out that strokes come in two main varieties: blockages and hemorrhages. A blockage can be either a blood clot or a vessel constriction (in combination with plaque that has built up on the internal walls of an artery). The oxygen can't get through to the brain, and the brain cells soon start to die for lack of fresh oxygen. A hemorrhage is an internally generated event in which blood vessels break or burst and sends blood out into and around brain cells. After a time, the blood-saturated brain cells die for lack of fresh oxygen.

My stroke was a hemorrhage. I'm told that because my natural ability to breathe and swallow had ceased by the time I got to the Emergency Room, one of the ER doctors had to manually help me breathe. I'm also told that the pain in my right leg grew so severe that I had to be sedated Sedation permitted other lifesaving efforts to go forward, including tests to provide a correct diagnosis.

The traditional reactive policy that most families follow—"you do what's best for him, and we'll sit by and pray"—is dangerous in this ever-more complicated world of health care. This is especially true in a life-threatening emergency, when the health care professionals diligently provide the services of their specialty (or subspecialty), but nobody is there to advocate the interests of the patient. Although the patient is not yet dead, in terms of making decisions he might as well be. So what does Paula—a just-retired federal executive—do when she finds herself in an ambulance with a body who used to be her husband? Of course, she gathers herself up and forms a research and management committee! It was called the "family stroke committee," and Paula ran it with the technical support of just one good cell phone, e-mail, four children, two sons-in-law, and two grandsons.

The family stroke committee engaged doctors and surgeons, nurses and hospital staff, and insurance companies in conversations— some of them desperate—about options on my behalf, together with assessments of risks, benefits, and costs. They addressed the issue of brain surgery along with a whole host of other serious issues that came at them in those first critical days and nights. And they gradually pieced together a family strategy, first for my survival, and then for my recovery and rehabilitation.

The surgery decision actually proved simple. The neurosurgeon who was called in on that Sunday morning to read the first CAT scan observed that the bleeding was too close to the vital expressive speech-communications network in the front-left lobe of my brain to risk surgery to relieve the pressure caused by the hemorrhaging. She also bolstered the family committee's resistance to the suggestion of another physician that my brain become the subject of a funded research study—something about testing a high-tech needle inserted through the cranium to withdraw the hemorrhaged blood. The needle would have to go right through the vital speech communications network, but he wanted to test it on me anyway. Even though we had not discussed the subject, Paula knew that I would have opposed any surgical procedure that would have run the risk of my being left alive but not able to take care of myself.

Ten years earlier my mother had suffered a hemorrhagic stroke. At the time, she was living alone in an Oregon beach community, and by the time they found her and moved her by helicopter to Portland, she was in even worse shape than I was a decade later. She had no living will or other advance directives, so the vital decisions fell on me as the oldest living relative. Paula knew how much I had wept and rued the day when, at the other end of a long-distance line to an ER doctor in Oregon, I failed to see my way with enough moral clarity to let him not feed her before she came out of the coma. Against the thinly concealed medical advice to let her die, I made the wrong decision. She lived for another nine years, never getting out of bed and having precious little relief from the mindless life to which she was committed.

Hence, when I slowly started functioning again, somehow I understood that Paula had made an affirmative judgment to keep me around a while longer. And from that day on, I wanted to prove that her decision had been the right one, and that I was going to come back to a full life.

Phase Two

It took five days of round-the-clock treatment in the intensive care unit (ICU) before the "wooze" started to wear off. I didn't exactly wake up, but Paula recalls the time when she squeezed my left hand and I squeezed back. I do remember being tied down to my bed so that I could not reach the tube in my mouth and tear it out.

Once I could breathe without it, I took stock and realized that although I was still alive, my mind and body were a shambles. My right side was paralyzed from my slack cheek and jaw down to my unfeeling toes. I had no control of my bodily functions, a fact that became clear when I discovered I could still smell. My vision, particularly on the right side, was impaired. I could hear all right, but I could barely comprehend what I was hearing. Worse still, I could not utter a syllable in response. I wanted to cry, in part to let my family know that I understood my sorry condition, but the tear ducts wouldn't work. Above all, I wanted to sleep—if I could bear the fragmented dreams about getting up and going back to work that my addled brain produced, in vivid color. But as much as I thought my body wanted it, sleep was the one thing that my family had to deny me.

Here we get into one of the most vexing characteristics of the "revolutionary" health care delivery system: the emergent role of insurance companies in prescribing patient care. It wasn't exactly that the hospital would deny me ER or ICU care without knowing who was going to pay for it, but the hospital was a lot more comfortable about

letting my care proceed when Paula had come up with my medical insurance cards. There was no question that the hospital could collect
its bills, but to get reimbursed it had to follow the guidelines provided
by the insurance companies.

One of the first things the family committee did was to ask my employer to send a copy of my entire primary insurance policy—not the
one summarized in the employee brochure, but the whole policy,
which runs more than 120 pages with amendments. It was important
to know as much as possible about the types of rehabilitation the policy would cover once I was out of ICU. Both the family committee
and my doctors believed that, because I was highly motivated and
marginally younger and stronger than many stroke victims, my best
chance to recover would lie in "aggressive rehabilitation" as an in-patient in a hospital that specializes in rehabilitation services. But this
strategy was going to be expensive, and my primary insurance company would have a thing or two to say about that.

My insurance policy provided "unlimited benefits for all covered
expenses" in a rehabilitation hospital, but there was a cap of 120 days
each calendar year for rehabilitation through a skilled nursing facility.
Representatives of my insurance carrier at first told my family and
hospital care providers (e.g., social workers) to limit our research to
local skilled nursing facilities with a less aggressive (and less costly) rehabilitation program. But my family and doctors relentlessly documented why aggressive rehabilitation was appropriate for me.

Paula and Jenna had determined that the National Rehabilitation
Hospital (NRH), located in northeast Washington, was one of the
highest-rated hospitals for the therapies that we needed. After visiting
NRH, they came away with an appointment for an NRH committee
to interview me at Fairfax Hospital, in order to determine whether I
had "the capacity to benefit" from the desired therapies for at least
three hours a day to start.

The next thing I knew, every time I would settle into what I felt
was badly needed sleep, it seemed that another member (or two) of
the family committee was there to awaken me, struggle to get my
limp body out of bed and into a wheelchair, and run me around the
hospital while talking up a blue streak to keep me awake. Well, it
worked! We demonstrated to the visiting NRH committee that I
could stay awake for at least three one-hour periods, and one day
later, I was on my way.

Phase Three

In-patient treatment at NRH is a 30-day boot camp for stroke patients. The morning after I got there, November 4, 1995, I was fed breakfast by a nurse who insisted that I would go hungry the next day unless I could use my left hand to eat. Then I was out of bed, into my wheelchair, and, just like that, wobbling but actually standing up under the physical therapist's support and watchful eye. Then I dragged my right leg through a few tentative steps before slumping to rest in my wheelchair. The regimen continued as follows: Back to bed for instant sleep, then into my wheelchair again and downstairs to spend an hour in occupational therapy (OT), trying to figure out what to do with my right arm It dropped like a rock when it fell off the wheelchair tray.

Lunch, bed, back into a wheelchair, sitting across from a speech therapist, trying to keep my eyes open and trying to answer her "capacity" questions by pointing at pictures so that she could find an entry point and begin building a rehab plan. I knew practically nothing, not even my name. Bed again. Get up for dinner, with family trying to help. Trying to say words like "love" and "good night" without success because of my puzzled brain and the incessant demands of sleep. (Beautiful was the first polysyllabic word that I could ever hang onto, months after graduation from NRH boot camp. Very slowly, but proudly, I told Pau-la that she was bea-u-ti-ful. This was true. And we both cried a lot. By that time, my tear ducts were working.) I was still pretty woozy during my first week at NRH. I didn't know whether I was comprehending anything until my stepson Brad broke through in a nice way. There were no weekend therapies, and so he drove over to NRH to break the loneliness very early Sunday morning. Saying that he wanted to resume betting on the slate of Sunday NFL games, something we'd been doing for years, he started going down the list of games and USA Today point spreads. He alternated the assignment of his picks and mine. But when he got to the big San Francisco-Dallas game, I suddenly pointed to the 49ers. Something told me that I wanted them to win because they were the team of "Hurryin' Hugh" McElhenny and Y. A. Tittle that I'd grown up with in Oregon 45 years ago, when San Francisco was the closest NFL team.

When Sunday visiting hours arrived, I somehow made it clear to Paula that I wanted to watch that game on television. We watched with no sound, so that she and others could talk. When the half-time score showing the 49ers ahead of the Cowboys flashed on the screen, I let out a loud "Yeah!" In that instant, Paula knew that my impaired vision had improved to the point that I could make out words and numbers, and, more important, that I could read them and they had meaning! She often says that this was a moment that she will never forget, even if it was football!

Once I began to comprehend what was happening around me, it was hard not to become frightened by my situation. I dreamed incessantly about going back to work. (What else is new, when you have believed for 30 years that success at work is the only true source of self-esteem?) On more than one occasion I was jolted awake in the middle of the night by the thought that I was alive, yes, but really good for nothing.

By the time day broke I was all right again, because there was something so magnificently simple about my whole situation. No phone messages to return, no meeting to attend, no plane to catch, no mortgage bill to pay. Just go to physical therapy (PT) and make my leg work to stand up and to walk; go to OT and make my arm work to squeeze or lift or type something; go to speech therapy and make my brain and voice work on one-consonant/one-vowel sounds like "ba" or "ca"; and see family and friends in visiting hours and make them feel comfortable. Sometimes I almost felt a sense of relief, because, in a curious sense, even though I was in the hospital, I was back in charge of myself. But of course I surely didn't control my hospital life. For a man suddenly rendered almost mute, who had shown control-freakish behavior from time to time, the most frustrating thing now was the interminable waiting. Sometimes I waited an hour in my wheelchair beside my bed before a nurse could break away from other more pressing duties to get me back into bed after a therapy. Twice I became so frustrated I tried to make the wheelchair to-bed transfer myself—whereupon, of course, I went sprawling on the floor.

After 10 days at NRH, Paula and my NRH neurologist arranged a conference call for all members of the family committee around the country. It fell to Jack to ask the really tough questions that everyone (including me) had been dancing around. These were, "What's the prognosis?" and "What should we and Dad be prepared for, long term?" To which my neurologist replied, in essence, keep your hopes up, but not too high—lest you be disappointed. Probably the mending of some of these injuries will be incomplete, and you (and he) will have to live with some sort of "condition" to be worked around as part of what otherwise can be a very good and rich and perhaps even long life. But he (and you) will have to work at it for a long time to make certain that it's the smallest and least intrusive "condition"—far beyond what we can do here at NRH.

But I equated "condition" with death, so I persuaded myself that my injuries were transient. I learned to walk clear around the atrium with only a cane and a physical therapist or a family member beside me to protect me from falling. I practiced going up and down stairs, one stair at a time. I learned to use my arm again, reviving and building up the shoulder, arm, wrist, and finger muscles.

When I was alone, however, I fell to wondering whether my right side would fully function again, whether I would have trouble avoiding incontinence, and whether my organs now served exclusively for liquid elimination would work for other purposes. Most of all, I wondered whether I would be able to speak naturally again.

At the same time, I became aware that Paula was going home every night after visiting hours to wrestle with a boatload of insurance forms and household bills and the boat was about to sink because I had neglected to make any provisions in advance for her to get to my funds. Fortunately, one night a practical-minded family friend simply handed me a pen to make my left-handed scrawl that would pass for my signature, and witnessed it—whereupon Paula could access my funds to pay our mounting bills.

On Saturday, December 2, 1995, I was released from the hospital. Of course I had to walk the minute I was outside the door. I was so happy to be alive, but just to be safe, we had a wheelchair in the back of the car.

Phase Four

It was obvious to everyone (except perhaps me) that I was going to be in for a long period of rehabilitation as an outpatient. After several hard winter months, during which Paula became exhausted from having to chauffeur me to NRH for my three outpatient therapies plus regular doctors' appointments, I gradually improved and the frequency of PT and OT slackened. We recruited two retired friends to handle the twice-weekly driving for my ongoing speech therapy, and left leaving Paula to do what she needed to do for her own rehab—yes, family members also need rehabilitation!

Meanwhile, it was getting increasingly difficult to pay for medical services, or any other kind, because I had used up my accrued vacation and sick leave and my short-term disability insurance benefits. It was time to face up to the grim fact that I was going to have to go on long-term disability insurance. I had paid absolutely no attention to this part of my employee benefits, and I hadn't focused on the choice I had made to limit my long-term disability insurance to 60 percent of my base salary. Nor did I understand that the insurance company's responsibility was only to make up the difference between my Social Security Disability (SSD) entitlements and 60 percent of base salary. Because of no provision for bonuses, the net result of these disability insurance arrangements was a reduction of my income not by 40 percent but by 75 percent! One other point. I guess it makes sense for long-term disability insurance companies to require you to get SSD benefits and deduct the amount of those benefits from the face value of your policy, but once you opt to receive SSD benefits, then you must live by the SSD rules and regulations. Simply put, SSD precludes you from earning even one dollar of personal income, on penalty of losing all of your SSD benefits. Because of the way the system is set up, being forced to claim your SSD benefits has a strong tendency to make you forever disabled.

I continued trying to be a hero. The Saturday I got home, Jack took me over to the high school track, and I ran around it twice before slipping back to a walk. After a while Jack took a picture of me resting on a track hurdle—leaving the distinct impression that I had been running and jumping hurdles on the same day that I was released from the hospital. I was touched when the picture came back to me as Jack's Christmas gift, with the inscription "No Hurdle Is Too High," however, I was encouraging family members to share my belief that, sometime soon, I was going to be back to my old self. That frightened Paula particularly.

I was determined to see our grandsons in New York, and sure enough, on January 12, 1996, while walking on a snowy Manhattan street carrying two sacks of groceries, I had a seizure. Fortunately, Paula had sent son-in-law Kevin out to find me when I wasn't back from the grocery store on time. He was with me when I went down and kept me from conking my head on the pavement. He helped me into an Indian take-out restaurant ("Curry in a Hurry") and called for an ambulance. Once again, I had driven myself beyond good sense, and my penalty was to spend a long, contentious, and frustrating weekend in a New York hospital. This disastrous experience had four effects:

First, I could not get released until I submitted to that miserable magnetic resonance imaging machine, in which my whole body was rolled horizontally into a space roughly the size of a Pringle's Potato Chip tube. I had to lie there perfectly still for an hour or so, fighting claustrophobia, while the technicians fired imaging beams into every part of the brain's affected area. Now I was sure that the cure was worse than the disease, but I survived. Fortunately, they found no further damage to my brain.

Second, I had to add a three-times-a-day antiseizure medication to my already burgeoning regimen of drugs and vitamins.

Third, and most disastrously, under the laws of Virginia, my state of residence, the privilege of being licensed to drive had to be further deferred for six months from the date of the seizure.

Fourth, and by far the most important, I had to spend three days thinking about how to work my way out of this mess, and that was a strikingly healthy development. Maybe I was going to have to stop kidding myself about going right on as though nothing serious had happened.

Aphasia/Apraxia

I had never heard of aphasia or apraxia before my stroke, but they are medical parlance for what was, and is, terribly wrong with my speech. Aphasia covers all kinds of brain-injury-related communications disorders that usually affect speech (expressive) and understanding of speech (receptive). The ability to read and write may also be reduced as a result of the brain injury. Apraxia is the term for a motor control disorder that involves the connection between my brain and the neurons that carrying messages of how to form words to my tongue, mouth, and jaw. As the June 1998 poster for Aphasia National Awareness Week put it, it's "when your brain holds your words hostage." I generally know precisely what I want to say; I just sometimes cannot say it.

My problem goes back to the hemorrhaging in the left-front lobe of my brain. The hospital CAT scan showed that was heaviest in the area

of my expressive speech-communications network. T hat was where
the brain cell died. I had to start learning speech almost from the beginning, "rewiring" my whole expressive speech function. My principal speech pathologist at NRH was a real professional who kept
working with me, trying various approaches, and steadily pushing me.
Finally I believed that I could never give up either. She also cured me,
finally, of evading my essential condition as a recovering stroke patient. One bright spring day in 1996 I went wheeling into her office to
announce that I had been invited to the annual North American
meeting of my management consulting firm, set for September.
Wouldn't it be a good idea for us to speed up our efforts so that I could
meet friends from the firm at the September meeting? No, she said. I
was flabbergasted, and asked, Why not? Because, John, you're not going to be ready by September, maybe not even by next September,
perhaps never.

I bolted from her office, onto the street, around the NRH campus,
crying uncontrollably. Twenty minutes later I was back in place, and
we were working on "tr" blends, as in "tree" or "train wreck," or
"truth." Later we laughed about it, sort of, but we both knew that she
and I had passed another milestone in the long march back from my
stroke. We had finally dealt not just with my symptoms but with the
workaholism. I understood that my efforts to get back to the lifestyle
that had been the underlying cause of my stroke had continually im-
peded my recovery and rehabilitation.

The Next Step

Soon after our spring epiphany, my speech pathologist began talking
to me about undertaking the next step in a university setting. The fact
is that I had become dependent on the speech pathology unit at
NRH, where I could speak just as I was able to and have listeners eager to help communicate with me. After more than a year, it was my
security blanket to ward off the outsiders who, because of my still-fal-
tering speech, would too often conclude that I was psychologically ill
or mentally retarded.

So, in the winter of 1996-97, 1 was transferred to the George Washington (GW) University Speech Center. Under the capable and insis-
tent guidance of the clinical director, usually hiding behind the
one-way glass of the clinical speech rooms, the graduate student-ther-

apists teach us dozens of strategies to make us more comfortable as we go about our lives, managing our disabilities rather than having to manage our frightful isolation. For example, we practice how to put a receptionist or a store clerk at ease by somehow explaining, "I can't speak because I've had a stroke, but if you'll bear with me, we can do some business." Now try that on the telephone!

Some Lessons

If you suspect that you might be a good candidate for stroke, ask yourself these questions: Are you overscheduled more often than not, so that time becomes a buzzsaw of hurry and worry, and time at home is just an overnight interruption of the important things you've got to do? Do you really like your work, or did something get off the track back there, and now it's a string of "gotta-dos" and "gotta-don'ts"? How many times a week do you feel stress or anxiety? I felt it every single day, and one day it just wore me out. You know that exercise reduces stress, but can you break away from work? Exercise can also help reduce blood pressure and weight, if either of those is a problem, but do you ever take time to check your pulse, weight, and blood pressure, or have your blood drawn and checked for cholesterol? And what do you eat, drink, or smoke? When you fail to control these fundamental health factors, you become a strong candidate for stress that can put you down, maybe for the count. My weight and cholesterol were on the high side, I exercised erratically (mostly when suddenly trying to lose weight), and my blood pressure had a tendency to "spike up" for no apparent reason, except maybe the presence of work-related stress.

If your family has a history of stroke, your risk for a stroke is a given, and you'd better adjust the basic work and health factors in your favor. At least you can make certain:

- That you and your family know what to do in the event of stroke-know the symptoms, the closest hospital with good stroke treatment, and the ambulance service that you can rely on to respond within 10 minutes;
- That you and your family select the best health and medical insurance that your employer(s) can offer and you can afford and that you have reference copies of your entire medical policies,

together with standing orders to send you all amendments as
they are issued;

- That you and your family purchase the most comprehensive disability insurance that your employer(s) can offer and that you
can afford;
- That your spouse or significant other has complete and immediate standby authority to get to (a) family financial resources, (b)
your medical records, and (c) the historical medical records of
your blood-relation family members; and
- That you and your family think about advance medical directives
and codify them in some kind of a living will.

So what else have I learned, other than that I would rather not have
had this experience? I have learned that after a stroke, life can never
be the same again, but if the injuries are not too severe, you can have a
second chance to build a new life—perhaps better than the first one
that you are forced to give up. I have learned that I was enormously
fortunate. I 'm told that there was a moment on that first Sunday
morning, when the ER doctors and nurses had done everything they
could, that less than an hour remained in my life unless somehow the
bleeding stopped in my brain. Not only did the bleeding stop but after
all the recovery and rehabilitation efforts spanning three years, almost
all of my receptive and expressive senses have returned. When I walk
around the GW campus, nobody knows I've had a stroke except when
someone stops me to ask for directions. And I have finally learned the
importance of family. As distracted a workaholic as I was for years and
years, I just didn't deserve the outpouring of love and support from
my family. But I'm going to take it, with exceeding thanks, and try to
live up to it in this new life.

The stroke, and everything that's happened since then, has taught
me the importance and the value of patience. In the hospitals, in the
therapies, and at home, it's the value that steels the courage to go on.
Impatience leads to frustration, and those two emotions simply upset
things. And in this new life, as the clinical director of the GW Speech
Center says, "maintenance is progress."

I have learned respect for "ordinary" people. I didn't recognize it at
the time, and I fought it every inch of the way, but in one blinding instant when I was stricken by stroke, I suddenly joined their ranks. All
of my influence and power, and three-quarters of my earning power,

were instantly drained away. And you know what? I certainly would not have chosen the route, but I kind of like being an ordinary person. There are more real people here. We make our own brand of very human respect, helping and being kind to one another. Being a power person is like a bad dream for me now.

In September I celebrated my 60th birthday with family and friends—including recovering stroke patients and therapists who have befriended me—and I went back to "speech school" at GW, beginning each week with the Monday morning stroke group. It always gives me hope.

Nate, Nan, and Never Say Die
Nate Berger

At age 46, without a care in the world, Nancy got hit with stroke. Actually, multiple strokes, on both sides of her brain. Perhaps as many as six strokes over a period of a few weeks. When she was finally medically stable, she was left with the thinking and reasoning ability of a three-year old child. We were told she would never get any better. Short of putting her into an institution, one of the options the doctors discussed with me; I was told to set her in front of a television set and hope for the best. She was only 46.

I was angry with the doctors who had given us such an evaluation, because, through no one wants to build on false hope, no one has the right to take real hope away from you. I told them they had no business predicting such a grim future for Nancy. First, they did not know how dedicated she could be to her own rehabilitation. Second, they had no idea of how devoted I was to improving her condition. And finally, they certainly had no idea of how much God loves us and would help us find a way past this situation.

In his prophetic song, "The Gambler", Kenny Rogers sings these words: ". . .every hand's a winner, and every hand's a loser, and the best that you can hope for is to die in your sleep." Here is how I interpret his words: In contract bridge, all the cards are dealt so that all teams around the room are playing the same hands. Everyone is the same. Some teams will struggle and barely make their game; some teams will not even do that well-not only do they not make their contract, they get hit with a penalty to boot. And then there are some teams that will not only make their game, but do so well they earn bonus points! Remember, they are all playing the same hands. Some just play it better than others. Certainly skill plays an part in this, but I think that most important consideration is ATTITUDE. With the attitude that you can win—you will! Besides deciding we were going to win, that is get the very best out of the life we had left, I also made up my mind that I would do anything and everything I could to make the best of Nancy's life as enjoyable and meaningful as possible. Certainly, unlike the Gambler, we could hope for more than just dying in our sleep!

I decided to use computers to help rewire Nancy's brain. Although now commonplace, in the '80s, personal computers were not yet in vogue. Few computer programs were designed for non-business needs. I had to adapt many of the programs that were available, but at least we had something. We got reading and spelling programs, and we would "play" together at the computer while she learned to add, subtract and read again. To rebuild her ability to think and reason, I got programs in analogous thinking. We used simple puzzles and games to develop problem solving skills, and I would scour catalogs of software programs for new sources to add as Nancy's skills increased. We also got a child's word processor program which she could use to keep a daily journal for herself. Because her short term memory was so poor, I asked her to write up each day the following morning, thus stretching and exercising her memory. As she progressed, she began writing to friends on her word processor. This allowed her to continue to interact with the real world, something many stroke veterans find themselves unable to do. But more importantly, Nancy had always been the person others would come to for advice. By writing letters, she was able, once again, to offer advice and help others. One cannot calculate the value of this to Nancy's self-esteem.

Throughout these experiences, I always stretched her and allowed her to use whatever skills she had. But I was careful not to let her become frustrated or dis-spirited if there were activities she could not do. For instance, she could not power up the computer by herself, so I installed a special program that would automatically start up in her journal program after she turned the computer on. Since she had the use of only one hand, she could not capitalize her words; she also concentrated so hard on getting her thoughts written that she often paid no attention to spelling or punctuation. No Big Deal! I simply went over her work after she was finished and "cleaned it up" so someone could read and understand it. It is a team effort, all the way, and we always had fun!

To prevent her body from becoming weak through inactivity, Nancy has several exercise programs she works at each day. For example, she rides an exercise bike 8 miles, in 32 minutes. Of course, she didn't start at that level. We began by having her ride for two minutes each morning, and I gradually increased the time she was on the bike. Over the course of several years, we got to the present level. There's no hurry—we have the rest of our lives. We can laugh about it now, but when we started, she once refused to do the bike. I told her that was okay, I simply wouldn't feed her dinner! "You can't do that!", she exclaimed. "No?" I asked. "Who are you going to report me to?" To keep her from getting bored, I read to her while she rides, then we can discuss whatever we have read while she was on her bike. Usually, we get the books that Oprah Winfrey recommends. If she has seen someone on T.V. who has written a book, we can get that, too. Both of us enjoy travel, and since Nancy's strokes, we have been to 27 countries on 6 continents. Nancy has been on the Great Wall of China, has been in a submarine exploring the Great Barrier Reef. She has been to the Vatican in Rome, the great cathedrals of France, the wonderful mosques in Morocco. We have been up the fiords in Norway, and rafted down rivers in the United States. Has it been fun? For Sure!! Has it been easy? Well, that's a different question. I give tremendous thanks to those who have gone before us. Others on crutches or wheelchairs who have forced a complacent society to pay attention to the special needs of people who can't do all the things most of us take for granted. An though the world has certainly become easier for the physically challenged person to get around, still, there is little traveling Nan could have done by herself—it is simply too hard. But we travel with the attitude that there is a way to do whatever it is we want to do, within reason. . . . We've had to give up hang gliding and pole vaulting, but to tell the truth, I'm not much for pole vaulting anymore anyway. But there are people who will help me carry her onto the boat for a Li River cruise in China. There are people who will help me get her into a horse-drawn carriage for a ride around Central Park in New York. Wherever we are in the world, there are many people who are more than willing to help. Trouble is, most of them simply do not know what to do. And many of us caregivers are not used to asking for others to help us.

Ask for help and let others help solve your problems. Nothing says you have to do it alone. My task, and the task of every caregiver/companion, is to figure out what needs to be moved, modified, changed, repositioned, added, eliminated - or whatever it takes to allow us to do whatever it is we want to do, within reason. . . . A good example: Bathrooms are a real problem for us. Often Nan has to get up in the middle of the night and transferring into the wheelchair and getting her to the bathroom is exhausting for the both of us. By the time she has finished, we are wide awake and neither of us can get back to sleep. Solution: I kicked myself for not thinking of this earlier. I bought a portable camp toilet—basically a folding pair of legs to which you attach a toilet seat and a disposable plastic bag. Got it at a sporting goods store for less than $20.00. We pack it in our suitcase, and set it up in the hotel room, right by Nancy's side of the bed. When she gets up during the night, we simply transfer her to the portable toilet, she does her thing, then we both get right back into bed and back to sleep. You've heard about working smarter, not harder?

Finally, this: Earl Nightingale tells the story of a farmer who found a pumpkin seed one day, and poked it into an Aunt Jemima syrup jug, filled the jug with dirt, watered it, and set the jug in a bright window. In a short time, the seed grew into a pumpkin, exactly the size and shape of the jug it was in. An Aunt Jemima pumpkin. Although the seed had the capability of growing much larger, it was held back by the container the farmer had put it into. People do the same thing with their lives. They poke themselves into jugs and then are forced to accept the limits of the jug—they can't grow beyond the boundaries of the container they put themselves into. There is no need to do that. Everyone has trouble in their lives. All of us sometimes feel we are lugging around more of a burden than we can bear, but Nancy says that God never puts more weight on you than he thinks you can carry, so get on with it. I wouldn't swap our troubles or defeats for someone else's. And I wouldn't trade our blessings and triumphs for anyone else's either. The days of our lives are, in the words of The Gambler, like the cards we have been dealt. And this is the hand we must play. I want to be certain that our hand is a winner! If you live your life with faith in God, don't ever lose hope, allow your mind to soar with inspiration, and keep the attitude that you can do whatever it is you put your mind to, all that you seek will be yours.

Craig and Carol: Stroke is a Family Illness
Craig Robertson and Carol Robertson

Testimony Presented to the Agency for Health Care Policy and Research

At this writing, C.R., a 37-year-old stroke patient with aphasia, was nearly 1 year post onset. His stroke recovery has been surprising in its breadth and depth. His initial status was severe in all vital spheres. He could not walk, talk, bathe, or toilet. The prognosis was fairly grim for such a bright young man with a wife and two children. He desperately wanted to get better and at the onset was assertively a part of the team's planning implementation process. He moved from yes/no question and a single communication book, then later to an alphabet board and finally to where C.R., an avid sports fan, employs internal coaching to arrive at his message and intent in a complete, coherent, and cogent manner. Four days per week, he puts into practice the above mentioned coaching model in his work reentry as a customer service agent for a major U.S. airline. One day per week he attends a vocationally driven rehabilitation program, where the physical therapist, occupational therapist, and speech-language pathologist review and refine the prior week's successes and debrief and detail the failures to ultimately ensure success so C.R. can resume his highly competitive job.

The Agency for Health Care Policy and Research (AHCPR) has as its mission to promote improvement in clinical practice and patient outcomes through more appropriate and effective health care services; to engender improvements in the financing, organization, and delivery of health care services; and to increase access to quality care. On June 12, 1992 its expert panel held a hearing on clinical practice guidelines on post stroke rehabilitation. The only consumer (person with stroke) to address the panel was C.R., whose poignant and prophetic testimony was as follows:

Craig's Story: Advocacy

My name is C.R., I am 37 years old and had a stroke in June of 1991, which left me with a right sided paralysis and severe aphasia. I am

here today during national Aphasia Awareness Week to talk about
stroke after the fact, particularly for those folks with aphasia who
might be unable to talk. The National Aphasia Association has asked
me to talk to you about my stroke and continued recovery nearly 1
year later. Last year, I could not say a word. Today, I'd like to say a
word about stroke.

The biggest problems for me after the stoke were not the physical,
but the stroke's impact on me and my family, on me and my friends,
on me and my job—it struck all of us and I'm still "recoiling." Stroke
actually is a lifelong recoiling, not a couple of weeks, or months, or
years—a lifetime of recoiling with my family, friends, and co-workers.
Everyday I am trying to realign my relationship with all comers—my
wife, my two boys, my friends, my employer. I will try to outline for
you three of the major problems that have happened to me this past
year and what I have learned from these experiences.

First, the emotional and psychological toll stroke takes on me and
my family is even more devastating than the financial toil. The fear,
the anxiety, the anger, all weigh heavily in the equation of rehabilitation. The necessary support, understanding, and therapy is at best uneven for many people with stroke. United, we tell all, that this is a
major concern—life daily requires persons with stroke to pay a penalty because of their handicap. Some stroke persons have more resources (rehabilitation team, family, community) than others. Policy
must recognize these areas of need and not limit or ration therapy to
weeks or months. Policy must regard potential for quality of life and
the ripple effect this will have on the family and community at large.

The second problem was work reentry. I am in my 30s and I want
to work. As I see it, the person with a stroke has four options: he can
return to his old job; he can return to his old company in a different
job; he can start a whole new job; or he can't or won't work.

None of these options are easy or attractive. All except the latter
may come after much work, money, and frustration have been ex-
pended. It seems that many roadblocks are in my way to becoming a
gainfully employed taxpayer again. The Americans with Disabilities
Act is not a solution but a tool. There must be a safety net that we can
cling to in this regard. Hope is my only hope.

The third problem is financial shock. The costs of stroke can be
said to be the cause of another stroke. They are very high in terms of
direct costs (health care dollars) and in terms of indirect cost (may not

be working). Typically a stroke survivor does not have the financial resources to go it alone. To recoil from the stroke, government must
provide additional spring—to cushion our fall and push us back into
the mainstream. I'm told that a dollar spent on rehab saves $9.00. We
must afford to invest in the potential of 2 million stroke survivors—a
million of whom have aphasia. The U.S. policy must be to strike back
at stroke by supporting its survivors and preventing such a trauma
from happening to others. Thank you for considering my testimony.

C.R. has not only returned to work, but as a result of his testimony,
he has hopefully helped to return the discussion of the clinical practice of post stroke rehabilitation to one with a face, a heart, and a
vision. C.R. and his remarkable continuing recovery of his communication skills is certainly testimony to the resilience of the human spirit
and the effectiveness of rehabilitation today.

Postscript: C.R. turns 40 next month. He has now been back to
work full-time as a customer service airline agent for nearly 2 years.
His performance appraisals have been outstanding—he has resumed
his leadership role in a highly complex and stressful work environment. He drives, parents, works, loves, and plays with renewed vigor.
He has resumed his avocation loves, boating and golfing, with adapted
equipment and attitude.

Carol's Story: Living With Stroke

I should start by saying that I'm not the person in my family who's had
the stroke. My husband Craig is. But I am certainly living with it, and
I am glad to have the opportunity to tell my story. A stroke does not
just affect the individual who suffers one, but all those around him or
her who are there to love and support him.

At 33, I was living the life I had always dreamed of. I had a loving
and supportive husband, two wonderful sons, ages 2 ½ and 5, and a
career I genuinely enjoyed. I had it all, until one sunny afternoon in
June when an aneurism in my husband's brain let go and he nearly
died while we were towing him behind our boat in an inner tube.
Thanks to the lifejacket he was wearing and the invaluable assistance
of my brother-in-law, we were able to quickly retrieve him from the
water and revive him. What we didn't know until a week later when I
found him disoriented and emergency surgery was performed, was

that the blood in his brain was causing the left mid-cerebral artery to clamp shut. On July 6, 1991, he suffered a massive stroke.

My life after that date was forever changed. Not only did I find myself having to deal with issues I never dreamed I'd have to face, such as the possible death of my 36-year –old husband and the father of my two boys, but such mundane things like where to take the car for repairs, and what do when the water heater lets go. We didn't have wills, and it now became an urgent issue that I have one, in case the unthinkable happened and I, too, suffered some calamity. My life that first month was a blur, and only seemed to get worse once Craig was released from the acute-care hospital directly to NRH. For the next two months, he underwent intensive therapy in an effort to

recover as much function as was possible, given the tremendous damage done by the stroke. When he arrived at NRH, he could no longer walk, talk, feed himself, or otherwise care for his personal needs. While everyone was positive and generous with their encouragement, the chances of Craig returning to a level of functioning that would allow him to return to work and the life we had did not seem particularly good.

I knew my first priority was to do everything possible to help Craig recover. He was clearly not accepting the "limited success" prognosis offered by the professionals, and he insisted that he would return to his old life and old job. If he believed that, then I had to also. Those two months of in-house rehab were exhausting for both of us. I spent early mornings with the kids and the housework, my days at work and evenings at the hospital with Craig. Most nights, I didn't get home until 11 p.m. I couldn't have done anything without our wonderful family, friends, and co-workers who all pitched in to help with the kids, the lawn, the house, and the jobs. The staff at NRH were equally fantastic. They responded to every question I had (and there were plenty of them) with knowledgeable, thoughtful answers, and never said "it can't be done." They included Craig in the treatment planning. They explained what was being proposed, even though they knew he couldn't speak. There were interim family meetings where Craig's NRH team each explained to me and our family where in the process he was. And, toward the end of his stay, there were the coveted "paroles" as we called them. These were days that I was able to take Craig out of the hospital, home for lunch or out to dinner with friends. Finally, just before Halloween, 1991, Craig was allowed to come home.

My desire to have life return to "normal" once Craig returned home was not to be realized. Craig's communication skills were still greatly impaired. He often could not find the word he needed, or would use the wrong word. "No" was (and is to this day) regularly mixed up with "yes." He had no use at all of his right arm or hand. His frustration resulted in angry outbursts at me and the kids. He had to reacquaint himself with how to use the microwave, the TV and the VCR. Of course, he was prohibited from driving. His judgment seemed to be dulled. He went out for a walk in the woods with the kids the first day home, and fell several times. The kids had to help him up. He tried to use the table saw and nearly cut off his good arm. It was as if he didn't fully comprehend the extent of his disability. His inability to drive was a tremendous inconvenience. This meant that I had to take him to appointments and therapy. He was always with me. What little "alone time" I had was gone. He even "stole" the car once to drive to the store; he thought no one would know. Finally, with help from NRH and specifically the OT staff, he got his provisional license.

As the months wore on, Craig improved little by little. Finally, in September of 1992, he returned to his old job as an operations agent for a large airline. Everyone at his company was wonderful, and often donated their own time to help him re-learn the voluminous codes and procedures necessary to do the job. Again, I thought my life would return to normal. Instead, this threshold brought with it a new set of challenges. His stamina was not what it once was, and he returned from work each day physically and emotionally exhausted. He'd sleep for a couple of hours, wake up long enough to have dinner, then go right back to bed. The kids, the laundry, the dishes, the bills all vied for my attention. What was worse, it seemed there was no one to take care of me.

Over time, I learned to carve out time for me. I developed a group of friends around the neighborhood, principally out of a need to because Craig no longer felt comfortable around most people because of his physical and speech deficits. I found my job to be a great comfort, mostly because it was the same as it had always been. When I walked through the door each morning, it was as if I was in a safe, predictable environment. We availed ourselves of the psychological counseling available through NRH. I can honestly say that I don't think I would have made it through those dark days without their help. We still go to see our "shrink," and probably will need to from time to time for the rest of our lives. I consider it an investment in my family's and my future.

I used to have dreams that Craig would walk through the door as he was before the stroke. I was obsessed with remembering him "before the accident." As time has passed, that has faded, so that now I have trouble remembering the "before." Is my life as I thought it would be? Yes and no. I wish this stroke had never happened, but there has been a great deal of good that has come out of it. I still have my husband and sons, and I believe I am much more sensitive to others needs, and infinitely more patient with people that I was before Craig's stroke. I try not to take anything for granted, because there's no guarantee it (or they) will be here tomorrow. While my relationship with my husband has changed too, my admiration for what he has accomplished against tremendous odds is greater than it ever was. I would never have chosen this path, but am grateful for what I have learned along the way.

Appendix A
Stroke Resources

- ABLEDATA
  8401 Colesville Road, Suite 200
  Silver Spring, MD 20910-3319
  (301) 608-8998 (V/TT)
  (800) 608-8958 (Fax)
  www.abledata.com
  An electronically maintained database of information on assistive technology that includes product description, prices, and contact information for product manufacturers.
- U.S. Health & Human Services
  Administration on Aging
  330 Independence Avenue, SW
  Washington, DC 20201
  (202) 619-0724
  www.aoa.gov
  Supports state and local programs for home-delivered meals, in-home assistance for the frail elderly, transportation services, legal assistance, employment help, and senior center programs.
- American Academy of Physical Medicine and Rehabilitation
  1 IBM Plaza, Suite 2500
  Chicago, IL 60611-3604
  (312) 464-9700
  www.aapmr.org
  A professional organization for physiatrists (specialists in rehabilitation medicine)
- American Association of Retired Persons (AARP)
  601 E Street NW
  Washington DC 20049
  (202) 434-AARP (2277)
  www.aarp.org
  The nation's largest advocacy group for senior citizens. Provides information and publications on safety, insurance, health care, caregiving, and long-term care.

- American Congress of Rehabilitation Medicine
  4700 W Lake Avenue
  Glenview, IL 60025-1485
  (847) 375-4725
  www.acrm.org
  A professional organization for rehabilitation professionals from a variety
  of fields.
- American Dietetic Association/National Center for Nutrition and
  Dietetics
  216 West Jackson Boulevard
  Chicago, IL 60606
  (312) 899-0040
  (800) 366-1655
  (900) 225-5267
  www.eatright.org
  Callers can be referred to registered dieticians or may listen to recorded
  messages on topics related to food and nutrition. The (900) number is
  staffed by registered dieticians; callers may ask specific questions for a
  charge of .95 per minute
- American Heart Association
  National Center
  7272 Greenville Avenue
  Dallas, TX 75231-4596
  (800) 242-8271
  www.americanheart.org
  Supports research, education, and community service programs aimed
  at reducing death and disability caused by cardiovascular disease and
  stroke.
- American Stroke Association
  7272 Greenville Avenue
  Dallas, TX 75231-4596
  (800) 553-6321
  www.americanheart.org/stroke
  Provides information and services for caregivers and people with stroke,
  including newsletters and other printed materials, stroke club support
  groups, and referrals to other resources.
- American Nurses' Association
  600 Maryland Avenue
  Suite 100 West
  Washington, D.C. 20024-2571
  www.nursingworld.org
  Professional organization for registered nurses. Sponsors the American

Nurses Foundation, American Academy of Nursing, Center for Ethics and Human Rights, and American Nurses Credentialing Center.

- American Occupational Therapy Association
  4720 Montgomery Lane
  PO Box 31220
  Bethesda, MD 20824-1220
  (301) 652-2682
  www.aota.org
  A professional organization for registered occupational therapists and certified occupational therapy assistants who provide OT services.
- American Physical Therapy Association
  1111 N. Fairfax Street
  Alexandria, VA 22314
  www.apta.org
  A professional organization for physical therapists and physical therapy assistants and students. Promotes the development and improvement of physical therapy service, education, and research.
- American Psychological Association
  750 First Street, NE
  Washington, D.C. 20002-4242
  (202) 336-5700
  www.apa.org
  Directs callers to the Psychological Association in their state for referrals to local psychologists.
- American Self-Help Clearinghouse
  Saint Clares
  25 Pocono Road
  Denville, NJ 07834-2995
  (973) 625-3037
  www.selfhelpgroups.org
  Provides callers with referrals and information for locating self-help groups. Also conducts training activities and publishes a self-help manual and a newsletter.
- American Speech-Language Hearing Association
  10801 Rockville Pike
  Rockville, MD 20852
  (800) 638-8255
  www.asha.org
  Provides callers with referrals to Speech-Language Pathologists who specialize in treating aphasia (ask for adult neurogenic communication disorders) and other specialties. Also distributes free and low-cost literature on a number of related topics.

- Children of Aging Parents (CAPS)
  1609 Woodbourne Road, Suite 302-A
  Levittown, PA 19057
  (215) 945-6900
  www.careguide.net
  A national clearinghouse for caregivers of the elderly who work in the
  field of aging. Provides information and publications about caregiving and
  support groups. Also provides referrals to other resources.
- CARF, The Rehabilitation Accreditation Commission
  4891 East Grant Road
  Tucson, AZ 85712
  (520) 325-1044
  www.carf.org
  Provides information on program accreditation. Send a self-addressed,
  stamped envelope and ask to receive a list of the accreditation rehabilitation facilities in your area.
- Consumer Information Center
  (Medicare information)
  Department 59
  Pueblo, CO 81009
  (719) 948-3334
  www.pueblo.gsa.gov
  A clearinghouse for booklets published by more than 40 federal departments and agencies. Established to help federal agencies develop, promote, and distribute consumer information to the public.
- Independent Living Research Utilization
  2323 South Shepherd, Suite 1000
  Houston, TX 77019
  (713) 520-0232
  (713) 520-5136 (TTY)
  www.ilru.org
  Provides brochures and publications about independent living, as well as
  a directory of independent living centers and organizations in the U.S.
  and Canada. Also offers technical assistance for independent living.
- Joint Commission on Accreditation of Healthcare Organizations
  One Renaissance Boulevard
  Oakbrook Terrace, IL 60181
  (630) 792-5000
  www.jcaho.org
  Accredits hospitals, home care facilities, ambulatory care facilities, long
  term care facilities, laboratories, and provider networks (HMOs,affiliated
  clinics, etc.).

- NARIC
  National Rehabilitation Information Center
  1010 Wayne Avenue, Suite 800
  Silver Spring, MD 20910
  (800) 346-2742
  (301) 495-5626 (TTY)
  www.naric.com
  A library and information center with over 50,000 references related to disability and rehabilitation; provides information and referrals to other resources.
- National Aphasia Association
  156 5th Avenue, Suite 707
  New York, NY 10010
  (800) 922-4622
  www.aphasia.org
  Provides information about aphasia, including a reading list, fact sheet, and newsletter; also refers callers to community-based groups and regional volunteer representatives.
- National Association for Continence
  P. O. Box 8310
  Spartansburg, SC 29305-8310
  (803) 579-7900
  (800) 252-3337
  www.nfc.org
  Provides health professionals and the general public with information about the causes, preventions, treatment, and management of incontinence.
- National Association for Hispanic Elderly
  1015 18th Street, N.W., Suite 401
  Washington, DC 20036
  (202) 293-9329
  Represents the interests of older Hispanics on issues such as income maintenance, employment, housing, support services, health care, and long term care.
- National Brain-injury Association
  105 North Alfred
  Alexandria, VA 22314
  (800) 444-6443 (Family Help Line)
  (703) 236-6000
  www.biausa.org
  Provides information about local NBIA chapters and support groups; also publishes a magazine and other materials for survivors of traumatic brain injury and their families.

- National Council on the Aging, Inc.
  409 3rd Street, SW, Suite 200
  Washington, DC 20024
  (202) 479-1200
  www.ncoa.org
  An advocacy organization representing the interests of older people and those who provide services for them.
- National Council on Disability
  1331 F Street, NW, Room 1050
  Washington, DC 20004
  (202) 272-2004
  www.ncd.gov
  An independent agency that provides leadership and recommendations for disability policy in order to promote equal opportunity and the full integration of people with disabilities in society.
- National Easter Seal Society
  230 West Monroe Street, Suite 1800
  Chicago, IL 60606-4802
  (312) 726-6200
  www.easter-seals.org
  An agency dedicated to increasing the independence of adults and children with disabilities. Provides information and printed materials.
- National Family Caregivers Association
  10605 Concord Street, Suite 501
  Kensington, MD 20895-2504
  (301) 942-6430
  (800) 896-3650
  www.nfcacares.org
  A not-for-profit membership organization that serves family caregivers; publishes a quarterly newsletter called *Take Care*! and runs a speaker's bureau.
- National Health Information Center
  P.O. Box 1133
  Washington, D.C. 20012-1133
  (800) 336-4797
  http://nhic-nt.health.org
  A federally supported information center that provides referrals for a variety of health- related matters.
- National Institute on Deafness and Other Communication Disorders
  31 Center Drive, MSC 2320
  Building #31 Rm 3C35
  Bethesda, MD 20892-2320
  www.nih.gov/nidcd

Provides free and low-cost materials about aphasia and other stroke-re-lated communication disorders; also conducts literature searches on re-search about aphasia and related disorders.

- National Institute of Neurological Disorders and Stroke
National Institutes of Health
31 Center Drive
Bethesda, MD 20892-2540
(800) 352-9424
www.ninds.nih.gov
The leading supporter of biomedical research on disorders of the brain and nervous system

- National Institute on Aging
Public Information Office
National Institutes of Health
31 Center Drive, MSC 2292
Bethesda, MD 20892-2292
(301) 496-1752
www.nih.nia.gov
Conducts and supports biomedical, social, and behavioral research on the aging process. Also distributes information and supports training activities and other programs related to aging.

- U.S. Department of Education
National Institute on Disability and Rehabilitation Research
400 Maryland Avenue SW
Washington, DC 20202-2572
(202) 205-8134
www.ed.gov/offices/osers/nidrr/
Supports national and international research for individuals with disabili-ties; sponsors a broad range of programs that focus on research and train-ing for researchers and clinicians, and distribution of new knowledge.

- National Stroke Association
96 Inverness Drive East, Suite I
Englewood, CO 80112-5112
(303) 649-9299
(800) 787-6537
www.stroke.org
Refers callers to local stroke support groups; also provides free and low-cost publications that are of interest to people with stroke and their families.

- President's Committee on Employment of People with Disabilities
1331 F Street, NW, Suite 300
Washington, DC 20004-1107

(202) 376-6200
www.pcepd.gov
Provides information, training, and technical assistance to business lead-
ers, rehabilitation and service providers, advocacy organizations, families,
and individuals with disabilities.

- Rosalynn Carter Institute
  Georgia Southwestern College
  800 Wheatley Street
  Americus, GA 31709
  (912) 928-1234
  www.rci.gsw.edu
  Focuses on the psycho-social difficulties and rewards experienced by families and professional caregivers who are helping people with emotional
  and mental problems, physical illnesses, and problems associated with aging.

- Visiting Nurses Association of America
  390 Grant Street
  Denver, CO 80203
  (303) 744-6363
  (888) 866-8773
  www.vna.colorado.org
  Develops competitive strength among community-based, not-for-profit
  visiting nursing organizations; works to strengthen business resources and
  economic programs through contracting, marketing, governmental affairs, and publications.

- The Well Spouse Foundation
  610 Lexington Avenue, Suite 814
  New York, NY 10022-6005
  (212) 685-8815
  (800) 838-0879
  A national, not-for-profit membership organization that offers support for
  husbands, wives, and partners of people who are chronically ill or have
  disabilities.

Appendix B
Rehabilitation
Program Checklist

The following checklist is designed to help you select a high quality rehabilitation program. When using this checklist, please note that it applies only to rehabilitation programs that provide *integrated* rehabilitation services (that is, programs that provide more than one kind of rehabilitation service in a *coordinated program of care*). Integrated programs include acute, subacute, day treatment, and outpatient rehabilitation programs.

How Do I Use This Checklist?

➡️ As explained above, the criteria in this checklist should *not* be applied to individual rehabilitation services that are not delivered as part of an integrated program of care, such as treatment at an outpatient clinic or in a nursing home where you receive only physical therapy, for example.

➡️ Except where specifically noted otherwise, the criteria in this checklist apply to all types of integrated rehabilitation programs (acute, subacute, day treatment, and outpatient programs).

➡️ For definitions and more information about the different rehabilitation programs and the services they provide, refer to the "Glossary" and the section of this guide titled "About Rehabilitation Programs."

➡️ Your doctor and/or medical social worker can help you use this checklist to choose the best program for your needs. Not only should they be able to answer many of the questions on this checklist (plus any other questions you may have), but they should also be able to refer you to other rehabilitation providers and administrators who can assist you.

➡️ Answer only those questions that apply to the type of rehabilitation program you are considering.

➡ In general, the more "Yes" responses to the questions in the checklist, the better the program. There is not a specific "grading scale" for this checklist. If it is helpful, you can make copies of this checklist and fill one out for each rehabilitation program you consider; that way, you can compare answers across programs.

The questions in this checklist are divided into four sections based on their importance. Each section should be evaluated as follows:

- **Section 1 - Meeting Industry Standards:** The questions in this section will help you determine whether a program meets standards set within the rehabilitation industry. Ideally, the program that you select should have "Yes" responses to all questions in this section.
- **Section 2 - Meeting Standards of Program Excellence:** The questions in this section will help you distinguish an excellent program from a good or average program. The more "Yes" responses to questions in this section, the closer the program comes to being an excellent, or "model," Rehabilitation program.
- **Section 3 - Meeting Your Personal Needs:** The questions in this section will help you determine how well a program meets your personal needs. You will want to have a "Yes" response for any of the questions in this section that are important to you.
- **Section 4 - Additional Considerations:** The questions in this section will help you determine whether the expected cost or duration of a particular program is likely to exceed any limits in coverage set by your health plan. They also provide additional points for comparison in evaluating similar programs. Please keep in mind that there are no rules or guidelines that can be used to judge a program as "good" or "bad" based on the responses to these questions.

Section 1
Meeting Rehabilitation Industry Standards

The questions in this section of the checklist are based on quality standards set within the rehabilitation industry. Accreditation is a status awarded to hospitals and other facilities that meet certain standards of excellence in their field. Programs that are accredited by CARF....The Rehabilitation Accreditation Commission have received a "stamp of approval" from professionals working within the rehabilitation field. Certification is a status awarded to facilities that are eligible to accept Medicare payments. Programs that are certified by Medicare must meet minimum health and safety standards.

Is the program accredited by CARF. . .The Rehabilitation Accreditation Commission?	☐ Yes	☐ No
Is the program certified by Medicare?	☐ Yes	☐ No
Has the program been in operation at least one year?	☐ Yes	☐ No
Does the program have a formal system for evaluating the progress made by all of its patients *and* the overall outcomes of the stroke rehabilitation program?	☐ Yes	☐ No
Are patients informed of their rights as they pertain to the rehabilitation program and facility?	☐ Yes	☐ No

For acute care and day-treatment programs:

Does the program offer a minimum of *three hours of therapy per day, five days a week*, and include services such as physical therapy, occupational therapy, speech-language pathology, social work, psychology, and therapeutic recreation, depending on your individual needs?	☐ Yes	☐ No

For subacute care programs:

Does the program offer a minimum of *one hour of therapy per day, five days a week*, and include services such as physical therapy, occupational therapy, speech-language pathology, social work, psychology, and therapeutic recreation, depending on your individual needs?	☐ Yes	☐ No

For all programs *except* integrated outpatient programs:

Does the program have a doctor available 24 hours a day, seven days a week, to respond to medical and rehabilitation needs?	☐ Yes	☐ No
Does the program provide the following additional rehabilitation services if they are needed?		
Audiology	☐ Yes	☐ No
Driver evaluation and training	☐ Yes	☐ No
Laboratory services	☐ Yes	☐ No
Nutritional services	☐ Yes	☐ No
Orthotics	☐ Yes	☐ No
Pastoral care/chaplaincy	☐ Yes	☐ No

Pharmacy services   ☐ Yes   ☐ No

Prosthetics   ☐ Yes   ☐ No

Respiratory care   ☐ Yes   ☐ No

Radiology   ☐ Yes   ☐ No

Rehabilitation engineering   ☐ Yes   ☐ No

Vocational rehabilitation   ☐ Yes   ☐ No

For integrated outpatient programs:

Does the program offer medical direction and therapy
provided by a doctor, and at least two other rehabilitation professionals (a physical therapist, occupational
therapist, social worker, speech-language pathologist,
vocational rehabilitation specialist, therapeutic recreation specialist, rehabilitation nurse, or psychologist)
who are selected based on your individual needs?   ☐ Yes   ☐ No

Does the program provide the following additional rehabilitation services if they are needed?

Audiology   ☐ Yes   ☐ No

Driver evaluation and training   ☐ Yes   ☐ No

Exercise   ☐ Yes   ☐ No

Medical Specialty Services   ☐ Yes   ☐ No

Nutritional Services   ☐ Yes   ☐ No

Orthotics   ☐ Yes   ☐ No

Prosthetics   ☐ Yes   ☐ No

Rehabilitation engineering   ☐ Yes   ☐ No

Sexuality counseling   ☐ Yes   ☐ No

Section 2
Meeting Standards of Program Excellence

The following checklist items are characteristics of "model," or excellent, rehabilitation programs, but are not necessary for CARF accreditation, or for
Medicare certification. These characteristics distinguish excellent programs
from good or average programs.

Is the program affiliated with other programs that offer rehabilitation services at other levels of care you

may eventually need (such as day treatment, outpatient treatment, or home care)?　□ Yes　□ No

Are the medical director and physicians who provide care in the program board-certified in physiatry or another rehabilitation-related specialty, such as neurology?　□ Yes　□ No

Does the program have on staff a full-time physiatrist (a specialist in physical medicine and rehabilitation) or another physician (such as a neurologist) who is experienced in rehabilitation medicine?　□ Yes　□ No

Is your personal physician welcome to visit you at the facility?　□ Yes　□ No

Does the program use a "team approach" in which the doctor, therapists, and other rehabilitation professionals work together and meet periodically to evaluate each patient's rehabilitation progress? (Note: Team conferences in acute, subacute, day treatment/CORF programs should be held weekly. Team conferences in outpatient programs should be held at least every 30 days).　□ Yes　□ No

Does the program hold "family conferences" to keep families up-to-date on the rehabilitation goals and progress of their loved ones?　□ Yes　□ No

Does the program have a stroke club or another support group for people with stroke and their families?　□ Yes　□ No

Does the facility host a consumer advisory group to seek input about its services for people with disabilities?　□ Yes　□ No

Does the program conduct home visits to make recommendations before discharging people who are returning home?　□ Yes　□ No

Does the program monitor the progress of individual patients by periodically measuring their functional ability and level of independence in activities of daily living (such as dressing and walking)?　□ Yes　□ No

Has the program implemented the "Clinical Practice Guidelines for Post-Stroke Rehabilitation" (published

by the Agency for Health Care Policy and Research in
May 1995)?   ☐ Yes   ☐ No

Section 3
Meeting Your Personal Needs

The following checklist questions relate to your personal needs, and are
among the characteristics you should consider in choosing a rehabilitation
program.

Is the facility convenient to family members and
friends who will be visiting?   ☐ Yes   ☐ No

Are the visiting hours of adequate length and at times
that are convenient for family members and friends
who will be visiting?   ☐ Yes   ☐ No

Does the program collect information from patients
and family members about their satisfaction with the
care they received?   ☐ Yes   ☐ No

If so, is the feedback generally positive?   ☐ Yes   ☐ No

Does the program participate in your health insurance
plan?   ☐ Yes   ☐ No

If not, will your health insurance plan cover any or all
of the costs of the program?   ☐ Yes   ☐ No

Will the program's staff assist with any paperwork re-
quired to make health insurance claims?   ☐ Yes   ☐ No

Section 4
Additional Considerations

There are no meaningful guidelines for evaluating your responses to the following checklist items. This is because what is considered a "reasonable" response for each of these questions will vary by both individual circumstances
(such as the age and health of the person receiving treatment, or their living
arrangement once they complete rehabilitation) and circumstances related
to the location of the program (such as the overall cost of living in the region,
the types of patients treated in the program, and the availability of alternate
levels of care in the area). However, these are questions you may want to ask,
particularly if you are comparing similar rehabilitation programs or evaluat-

ing the completeness of your health coverage, in terms of any limits that may exist on total costs or length of stay.

What is the program's "average length-of-stay" for people with stroke?

_____
days

What percent of people with stroke return home, rather than being placed in nursing homes, after discharge?

_____ %

What is the average total cost for the complete stroke program (acute rehabilitation, home care, outpatient)?

$_____

Managing Stroke: Additional Readings and Resources

Chapter Three: Health Insurance and Medical Rehabilitation

Resources

- Agency for Health Care Policy and Research
  Suite 600
  2101 East Jefferson Street
  Rockville MD 20852
  (301) 594-6662
  www.ahcpr.gov
- American Association of Health Plans
  Suite 600
  1129 20th Street, NW
  Washington, DC 20036-3421
  (202) 778-3200
  www.aahp.org
- American Association of Retired Persons
  601 E Street, NW
  Washington, DC 20049
  (202) 434-2277
  www.aarp.org
- Health Care Financing Administration
  (Medicare and Medicaid programs)
  7500 Security Boulevard
  Baltimore, MD 21244-1850
  1 (800) 638-6833
  www.hcfa.gov
- Health Insurance Association of America
  600 East
  555 13th Street, NW
  Washington, DC 20004-1109
  (202) 824-1600
  www.hiaa.org

- National Committee for Quality Assurance
  Suite 500
  2000 L Street, NW
  Washington, DC 20036
  (202) 955-3500
  www.ncqa.org

Additional Readings

DeJong, G., & Beatty, P.W. (1999). Managed care and neurologic injury: The case of stroke. *Topics in Stroke Rehabilitation;* 5(4):1-16.

Gottlieb, M. (1998). *The Confused Consumer's Guide to Choosing a Health Care Plan.* New York: Hyperion.

Chapter Four: Planning To Strike Back At Stroke

Additional Reading

Ozer, M.N., Payton, O.D., & Nelson, C.E. (1999). *Treatment Planning for Rehabilitation: A Patient Centered Approach.* McGraw Hill Inc.: New York.

Chapter Seven: Communication and Swallowing Problems

Additional Reading

Tanner, Dennis, (1999). *The Family Guide to Stroke and Communication Disorders,* Allyn and Bacon, Boston.

Chapter Nine: Quality of Life After Stroke

Additional Reading

Astrom, M., Adolfson, R., Asplund, K. (1993). Major Depression in Stroke Patients: A 3-Year Longitudinal Study. *Stroke,* 24(7): 976-982.

Bergquist, W. H., McLean, R. , Kobylinski, B.A. (1994). *Stroke Survivors.:* Jossey Bass Publishers, San Francisco.

Burrill, P.W., Johnson, G.A., Jamrozik, K.D., Anderson, C.S. Stewart-Wynne, E.G., Chakera, T.M. (1995). Anxiety Disorders after Stroke: Results from the Perth Community Stroke Study. *British Journal of Psychiatry,* 166(3): 328-322.

Heilman, K. M., and Valenstein, E., (1984) *Clinical Neuropsychology*, 2nd edition. Oxford University Press, New York.

Robinson, R. G. and Benson, D. F. Depression in Aphasic Patients: Frequency, Severity and Clinical-Pathological Correlations. (1984) *Brain and Language* 14: 282-291.

Sipski, M. L. and Alexander, C., (1997). *Sexual Function in People with Disability and Chronic Illness: A Health Professional=s Guide*.: Aspen Publishers, Gaithersburg, MD.

Sobel, D.S. and Orstein, R. (1996).*The Healthy Mind, Healthy Body Handbook*.: DRx, Los Altos, CA Tel. (415)-948-6293.

Stuss, D. T. and Benson, D. F. (1986). *The Frontal Lobes*.: Raven Press, New York.

Chapter 10: Technology and The Internet: A Convergence of High Tech

Resources

From month to month and even day to day, new things become available on computers, and many of them can come into your home or into your community library through the Internet, at no financial cost. Getting information from 'the Web' is something that you or your family member can do. It is easier, and often more effective, than looking for information in a book. The more you do it, the easier it gets.

But don't forget the most user-friendly source of information there is! Your community librarian can in moments help you to find almost anything, or at least show you where to look. The librarian knows what books, what magazines, what organizations, what regulations, and what services there are and where to find out about them. If you need help getting started on using the computer, libraries often have people to help you out. Please also refer to Appendix A for a host of other Stroke related resources.

- Amazon.com (www.amazon.com) has a good selection of books for and about people recovering from strokes. One easy way to get to this information is by typing in "one hand" under the search section.
- Kim, H. (Apr. 1999) "The long view: selling providers on telerehab," TeleRehab Report 10(4):15-19. An example of rehabilitation providers "visiting" stroke patients via telecommunications is discussed.
- Annual product review issues appear in magazines like *Rehab Report* (formerly *Team Rehab*) and *Advance for Directors* on technologies such as wheelchairs.

World Wide Web Sites

- National Stroke Association's homepage is at http://www.stroke.org. They can also be reached by phone at 800-STROKES (787-6537). This site provides stroke prevention, treatment, and rehab information. The organization produces the *Be Stroke Smart* newsletter for families and caregivers of stroke patients and the patients themselves. This site has dozens of links to products and services for stroke survivors and their caregivers. There are, for example, reading and writing aids, exercise equipment, lifts and ramps. The value of visiting this site is that it's a one-stop-shop and is stroke-specific.
- The Disability and Medical Resources Mall, at http://www.coast-resources.com. This site provides "electronic shopping" from your desk top. It will connect you to hundreds of product and service vendors.
- The American Heart Association, at http://www.amhrt.org. The American Stroke Association is part of this organization. Links from this site will connect you to other people with strokes and their families. You can also print out their newsletter from this site. American Heart Association Stroke Connection at 800-553-6321 provides educational books, videos, and tapes about stroke for patients and their families. It also refers to stroke clubs and other self-help groups.
- Web Med, at http://webmd.lycos.com. Enter the word "stroke" in the search area, press "stroke" and you'll be pointed to information on self care, and many other Internet links and support resources for more help and information.
- Intelhealth, at http://www.intelihealth.com. This is the Web site of Johns Hopkins Health Information. Enter the word "stroke" in the search area, press "stroke" and you'll be pointed to very easy-to-read information on rehabilitation, preparing a living place, deciding about special equipment, and other more useful information.

Technology Assistance for People Recovering from Stroke

- Tech Act projects in each state and territory provide information on living with disabilities. RESNA, the Rehabilitation Engineering and Assistive Technology Society of North America, has a contact list, which can be accessed by calling: 703-524-6686.
- National Easter Seals: 312-726-6200. Provides books, pamphlets, and audiovisual materials about disabilities and provides guidance about assistive devices such as wheelchairs. Via their "Easy Access Housing"

Internet page (www.seals.com), information is provided for making homes more safe and accessible.

- The Job Accommodation Network is a free service providing information regarding your rights under the Americans with Disabilities Act (ADA) and also possible accommodation ideas. Free literature is provided, as are free consultations with experts in the field. Obtain contact information at: 800-526-7234 or on the Web at: www.janweb.icdi.wvu.edu

- National Alliance for Caregiving: 301-718-8444. Has produced a volume titled *Family Caregiving in the U.S.*, 1997.

- Stroke Support Information Website at http:member.aol.com/scmmlm/mdin.htm is hosted by recovering stroke patients and has a wide range of information and resources for both stroke patients and their caregivers. It includes a chat room and an extensive list of books on stroke recovery that may be purchased online.

Professional Organizations to Call for Technology Assistance

The Association of Driver Educators for the Disabled (ADED): www.driver-ed.org or call: 608-884-8833.

Companies and Catalogs Offering Products for Daily Living

- Infogrip, Inc. Sells many assistive software and hardware devices via catalog, including: adapted keyboards, pointing devices (alternatives to the mouse), etc. The company can be contacted at: www.infogrip.com/ 800-397-0921.

- The Assistive Communication Products catalog from HITEC interprets "communication" very broadly and covers devices relating to phoning, alerting, remote control, and other at-home activities. Reach them at 800-288-8303 or www.hitec.com.

- *The Sammons Preston Enrichment Catalog*. This covers a variety of aids for self-care, home adaptations, and exercise. Call 800-323-5547.

- *Achievement Products for Seniors*. This catalog is roughly comparable to the *Sammons Preston Enrichment Catalog*. They can be reached at 800-373-4699.

- Maadak, Inc. manufactures aids for daily living. Their site is at www.maddak.com or you can call customer service at: 973-628-7600 to order a catalog. Other companies that also offer these items include

Sammons Preston, whose site is at www.sammonspreston.com or call: 800-323-5547; and North Coast Medical, whose site is at www.ncmedical.com or call: 800-821-9319.

- Parrot Software offers products for people with language and memory disorders and helps with reading and word finding. Call 800-727-7681 or write for a free catalog, at catalog@parrotsoftware.com
- *Sears Home Health Care Catalog, 1999-2000.* Call 800-326-1750 for a catalog picturing a range of products to assist in the home.

In addition, there is a range of sites offering specific products for specific disabilities, such as hearing or eyesight failure. See, for instance, The Lighthouse International site at www.lighthouse.org. There you can be directed to products for those with failing sight. For particular needs, such as computer usage by persons with disabilities, there is, for instance, the Center for Computer Assistance to the Disabled (CCAD) which has as its mandate enhancing the quality of life for people with disabilities through use of modified personal computers, adaptive devices, and customized software. The CCAD can be contacted at 214-800-2223 or on the Web at: www.c-cad.org Other companies produce products that can assist the disabled user, such as Dragon Systems, whose products offer the capability to speak to the computer to communicate rather than type. Their contact information is: 617-965-5200 or on the Web at: www.dragonsys.com

We also encourage you to also visit the Abledata Web site, at www.abledata.org. It lists more than 24,000 products from nearly 3000 companies. The listings include high-tech, low-tech, and "no-tech" products, in the database developers' own words. There is also a special page with resources for stroke and brain-injured patients. Click the "Stroke and Brain Injury" box after clicking on the "Resource Centers" entry on the home page. They note as well that the product listings include everything from adaptive clothing and canes to computer hardware and software to powered wheelchairs to chair lifts and grab bars. Check it out!

Glossary

accreditation: a status awarded to hospitals and other facilities that meet certain standards of excellence in their field

activities of daily living (ADL): routine activities a person does every day, such as standing, sitting, walking, eating, bathing, and grooming

acute medical care: medical care that is meant to stabilize one's medical condition and minimize complications; usually received before rehabilitation

acute rehabilitation: medical services that include both general medical care and medical rehabilitation services

allowable charges: the maximum amount the Medicare program or other health insurance plans will pay for particular healthcare services

aphasia: loss or impairment of the ability to express or understand spoken or written words

apraxia: loss or impairment of the ability to perform complex muscular movements

assistive equipment: equipment or devices, such as wheelchairs, braces, walkers, or speech aids that help a person to perform activities of daily living

balance billing: charges for doctor's services that exceed Medicare's allowable charges and for which patients are responsible, up to a predetermined limit

benefits: services or equipment that a health insurance plan will pay for

cap: a limit on the amount an insurance plan will pay for a person's health care each year, or over a lifetime

case manager: a professional who works for an insurance company, hospital, or rehabilitation facility to make sure that all aspects of treatment comply with the rules of an individual's health plan

catastrophic limits of coverage: under a health insurance plan, the maximum out-of-pocket expenses a person must pay for medical services or prescription drugs

certification: a status awarded to facilities that have met minimum health and safety standards and are eligible to accept Medicare payments

combination plan: a health insurance plan, such as a preferred provider organization (PPO), that combines features of both traditional indemnity policies and managed care plans

comprehensive outpatient rehabilitation facility (CORF): a rehabilitation facility that provides a full range of rehabilitation services on an outpatient basis

copayment: a small, fixed-dollar amount (usually $5 or $10) paid by the patient for a doctor's visit, prescription drugs, or other healthcare services

covered benefits: health care services that are paid for by an insurance company according to the health insurance policy

custodial care: care that is provided to help patients take care of their daily needs (eating, bathing, dressing, etc.) that does not require treatment or services from specially trained professionals, such as doctors, therapists, or nurses.

day treatment: rehabilitation care that provides a full range of intensive services, but allows patients to stay at home overnight

deductible: a dollar amount that the patient must pay before an insurance company begins paying for any services; the amount varies by insurance plan

disability: a problem with a human activities, such as not being able to walk

dysarthria: loss or impairment of the ability to produce speech

dysphagia: impairment of the ability to swallow liquids or solids

environmental adaptations: conditions or things in a person's environment that enhance independence, such as ramps or elevators

fee-for-service (FFS): a method of payment for medical services in which a specific fee is charged for each individual service; the method of payment used under traditional indemnity policies

functional ability: how well a person is able to perform activities of daily living (eating, bathing, dressing, communicating, etc.) without help from someone else

gatekeeper: a person at a health insurance plan, generally a primary care doctor, who approves treatment (and thus payment) for health care services, such as rehabilitation services

handicap: a problem caused by one's environment that limits participation in certain daily actives, such as steps that create a barrier for a person in a wheelchair

health maintenance organization (HMO): (see managed care plan)

hemiparesis: weakness in one side of the body

hemiplegia: paralysis on one side of the body

impairment: a physical problem with a body or organ function, such as paralysis

indemnity policy: a traditional health insurance plan through which the patient is treated by his or her choice of physician and pays on a fee-for-service basis

long-term care facility: (see nursing home)

managed care plan: a health care plan, such as a health maintenance organization, that delivers comprehensive health careservices at a reduced price for members who agree to use certain providers and facilities

Medical Hospital Insurance (Medicare Part A): a part of the Medicare program that covers medical treatment in a hospital, skilled nursing facility, or hospice, as well as medical care a person receives at home from a home health care service

medical social worker: a medical professional who helps patients solve problems related to their need for medical care by answering questions, providing information, offering counseling, and making referrals to other professionals and resources in the community

Medicare: a health care insurance program administered by the federal government that provides health insurance for people over age 65, some people with disabilities, and others who qualify

Medicaid: a health insurance program run by individual state governments that provides health coverage primarily for low-income families and people with significant disabilities

Medicare Part A: (see Medical Hospital Insurance)

Medicare Part B: (see Supplementary Medical Insurance)

medically stable: a medical term that means a person's condition is not likely to get worse or develop medical complications

Medigap policy: a health insurance policy purchased through a private insurance company that pays for medical expenses not covered through the Medicare program

neglect: the act of disregarding stimuli on the side of the body that has been affected by a stroke

network: a group of health care providers and facilities that participate in a managed care plan or preferred provider organization

neurologist: a doctor who specializes in diagnosis and treatment of problems with the nervous system

nursing home: a facility where patients stay to receive rehabilitation services, long-term care, or skilled nursing care

occupational therapist (OT): a rehabilitation professional who teaches skills and adaptations that allow people with disabilities to be as independent as possible in their daily activities

orthoses: devices designed to support or supplement a weakened joint or limb

out-of-network: providers and facilities that do not participate in a particular managed care plan

out-of-pocket expenses: the costs of healthcare services that the patient must pay because they are not paid for through an insurance plan. These include both copayments and deductibles.

outpatient rehabilitation: rehabilitation services provided to a person who lives at home; may be a comprehensive, daily program of multiple services, or only one or two services once or twice a week

paralysis: the inability to move a part of one's body, such as an arm or a leg

pastoral care: spiritual support and guidance provided by a chaplain, or other clergyman, to address the emotional and spiritual needs of rehabilitation patients, their families, and members of their rehabilitation team

physiatrist: a doctor who specializes in physical medicine and rehabilitation

physical therapist (PT): a rehabilitation professional who works to restore one's movement abilities

point of service option (POS): in a managed care plan, the option to pay a higher price for healthcare services in order to choose providers or facilities outside the plan's network

preferred provider organization (PPO): a health insurance plan that offers a discounted price for health care services to members who use approved (that is, Anetwork@) providers or facilities

primary care physician: a doctor who provides non-specialist medical care; primary care doctors often are responsible for referring patients to specialists if needed

prostheses: artificial limbs or body parts

quality of life: a person's level of satisfaction with all aspects of his or her world, including self-esteem, personal and family relationships, social activities, financial conditions, employment status, spiritual activities, and anything else that influences satisfaction with life

rehabilitation services: individual medical or rehabilitation treatments received as part of a medical or rehabilitation program. Rehabilitation services include medical and nursing care, laboratory tests, rehabilitation therapies such as PT or OT, counseling sessions, recreational activities, and anything else prescribed to increase a patient's independence

skilled nursing facility (SNF): a facility that provides patients with a high level of nursing care and meets certain industry standards

speech-language pathologist (SLP): a rehabilitation professional who works to restore communication and swallowing skills

stroke: a sudden interruption of blood flow to an area of the brain, caused by a blockage (a blood clot) or by bleeding (a cerebral hemorrhage).

stroke club: a local organization that offers programs and support for people with stroke and their families

subacute rehabilitation: rehabilitation services that include daily nursing services, supervision by a rehabilitation doctor, and medical care as needed; subacute rehabilitation is less intensive and generally lasts longer than acute rehabilitation

Supplementary Medical Insurance (Medicare Part B): additional health insurance coverage that may be purchased through the Medicare program by people who qualify for Medicare

transfer between levels of care: the movement of patients between different treatment programs and settings so that they may receive the most appropriate type of care

Index